How to Find Your Man Is Ideal for Lifetime Commitment?

The Complete Guide for the Women, who want to Find out the Ideal, Perfect and Loving Man for The Lifetime Commitment, when you Are in Love

By reading this document, the reader agrees that under no circumstances is the author responsible for any losses, direct or indirect, that are incurred as a result of the use of information contained within this document, including, but not limited to, errors, omissions, or inaccuracies.

Table of Content

Introduction

One of the human being's deepest needs is to love and be loved. Many people long for the warmth of a long-term romantic relationship where love can be shared. When there is love, a relationship is made and then commitment. This is important because a partnership has no conditions in which it works without liability and, therefore, cannot be held accountable either.

You're probably happy and excited when you think you've found the person you'd like to commit to forever. That phase in a commitment where you haven't discussed where you are yet, but you know that you're both secure and in love is one of the most fun times in a couple's life. While some confusion may still exist, which can make it even more exciting, there (hopefully) should also be a lot of happiness. But sometimes the solution might not always be that simple. You may be someone who values verbal affirmation of commitment over anything else, or perhaps the person you see with their emotions may not be forthcoming. And, maybe you're happy in a relationship and want a little more evidence that your partner is willing to engage with you. It's not uncommon to be sure that the person you love is dedicated to you.

All relationships are different, of course, and some people will vary in the way they show affection and commitment. You can make life-long sacrifices and promises to yourself and your spouse to commit yourself to your partner. You must able to dedicate yourself to your relationship with the will. Commitment is what holds an enduring marriage. It requires trust, energy, and integrity. It is the quality that allows the two people to support a healthy and robust relationship. Both partners must be willing to have equal sacrifices, time, and faith for commitment to play a decisive role in a relationship. Women are mostly found as an ideal man for the lifetime commitment. Here is a question of who is an ideal man? A man who is ready for the commitment will be according to your expectations. Every woman is found of an ideal man for the lifetime commitment with whom she spends her whole life happily. Lifetime commitment is not secure at all; you can say that Lifetime Commitment is about sharing, respecting, growing, and prospering with each other's commitment without any involvement in controlling, manipulating, invading, or abusing the other in any way. You have to spend your life with one person, and it's important to choose the right person for commitment. Who loves you, cares for you, understands you, and according to your expectations. This book is written primarily to teach women how to assess the ideal man committed to a lifetime. Using various techniques, you will learn realistic ways to find the ideal man. The book shows you how to find your man. Whether you're trying to capture the heart of your ideal man for keeping or you're only interested in flings, in this fantastic book, you'll find a tone of useful information.

This isn't a theory book, so be prepared to apply what you're about to read. The approaches I share in this book are time-tested techniques that have been accumulated over several years from the experiences of countless women. They work, but you have to be willing to do it.

Chapter 1

Ideal Man

An ideal man does not come from an ideal look norm. It's a perfect man, it is difficult to describe, but an ideal man is someone who has a beautiful soul and kind-hearted, who also has an inner strength. An ideal man should be a gentleman, not a prize; he should treat you like a lady. He loves you, and you would do the same thing.

He doesn't have to know what you do; he has to understand that you love him, and that's a plus if he likes it! He can listen, and he can tell you when you need his attention and willingly give it. An ideal man is in shape throughout the year, he is mindful of his looks, and he has a good sense of dress, trendy yet modest, and never found unkempt. An ideal man is self-assured, not allowing his insecurities to cloud his judgment, he is a brilliant conversationalist talking with intelligence, having a sense of humor, the ability to put a smile on your face and make you laugh, that would always give him the upper hand!

He's a friend of yours, your heart, and your encouragement. He is always there to talk to you, to correct you, and to console you, as well as to be emotional. He has faith in you and is trying to make you comfortable with physical strength.

Some Characteristics of an ideal man:

While the reasons we fall in love is a mystery, much less mysterious are the reasons we remain in love. It is possible that maybe no such thing as the ideal man but is someone who has established himself in specific ways that go beyond appearances and success can be found as an ideal man. Although we each pursue a different set of qualities that are special to us individually, there are certain psychological traits that both you and your partner should aspire to make the relationship much more likely to be successful in the long term.

A common criticism that people make of their partners is that they have to "grow":

How many of us are unaware of is that growing up is not just about behaving like an adult? Ultimately growing up means recognizing and overcoming failures in early childhood and then realizing how these incidents affect our current behavior.

The ideal man is, therefore, able to focus on their experience. They have a maturity that comes from their family of origin being emotionally emancipated. They also developed a strong sense of autonomy and freedom, making the mental change from boy to man or girl to female. Having broken ties with old identities and patterns, this person is more open to their partner and with the new family they have created, as opposed to the one they were born into.

Because this person has grown up, in an intimate relationship, they are less likely to re-enact childhood experiences. They are not looking for someone to compensate for flaws and weaknesses because they have matured as a human. They don't seek someone to complete their incompleteness. He's searching for someone like himself. They are searching for another person with similar qualities to theirs, with whom they can share their lives in a cooperative manner.

2. Open and non-defensive:

An ideal man is free and unprotected and willing to be vulnerable. As a result, without being overly sensitive to any topic, they are accessible and receptive to feedback. Their openness also allows them to express feelings, thoughts, dreams, and desires straightforwardly. This has a social and sexual development value

3. An ideal man is honest and lives with integrity:

In a close relationship, the ideal man realizes the importance of honesty. Honesty builds people's trust. Dishonesty confuses the other person with their sense of reality, destroying their confidence. Nothing has a more damaging effect than fraud and deceit on a close relationship between two men. The blatant deception involved is often more harmful than the unfaithful act itself, even in such painful situations as infidelity.

The ideal partner seeks to live a life of honesty to avoid inconsistencies between the words and actions of one. It extends to all interaction grades, both verbal and non-verbal.

4. An ideal partner is supportive of each other and receptive to each other, with unique individual ambitions and priorities:

Ideal man considers the interests of each other independently from their own. They feel comfortable with each other's overall goals in life and support them. They are sensitive to the needs, desires, and feelings of the other and put them with their own on an equal footing. Of dignity and empathy, the best couples treat each other. With threatening or manipulative behavior, they don't try to control each other. We value the distinct personal boundaries of each other while being physically and emotionally connected at the same time.

5. An ideal man has empathy and understanding of their partner:

The ideal partner perceives their partner at both an analytical, observational, and an intuitive, emotional level. This partner can understand their mate as well as empathize with her.

When a couple understands each other, they are mindful of their commonalities and consider and appreciate the differences. Each partner feels understood and validated when both partners are empathic, that is, able to communicate with feeling and respect for the desires, attitudes, and values of the other person.

6. An ideal man is physically affectionate and sexually responsive on many levels:

Physically, emotionally, and verbally, the ideal man is easily devoted and sensitive. They are personal, recognizing, and expressing warmth and tenderness feelings outwardly. We enjoy the closeness to being intimate and are uninhibited during lovemaking to freely give and receive affection and pleasure.

7. An ideal partner will have a sense of humor!

The ideal man is funny. A sense of humor in a relationship can be a lifesaver. The ability to laugh at own self and the weaknesses of life allows a person to maintain a proper perspective while addressing the sensitive issues that arise within the couple. Playful and teasing couples often with their humor defuse potentially volatile situations. The awkward times in a relationship are certainly relieved by a good sense of humor.

While some of us are more brain-like than others, smarter men are more likely to get married and remain committed, according to studies. You may have a guy on your hands that is more likely to be faithful.

8. An ideal man makes you laugh:

It's vital to find somebody with whom you can laugh-even if everyone else rolls their eyes at his father's jokes, though they crack you up, it's all essential.

9. An ideal man actively supports your career:

Man has been a decisive factor in two-thirds of women's decisions to quit their jobs; an ideal man will help you and assist you in all circumstances.

10. An ideal man makes as much effort with your friends and family:

It's not unusual for a woman to end up giving up her own social life to step into her new man's. But it's rare for a man to do the same once a relationship is entered.

This is ridiculous; in fact, it is essential to maintain your friendships. So make sure you're with a guy who not only encourages you to spend time with your mates but also seeks to get to know them.

11. An ideal man is emotionally smart:

If you want to believe in myths, it's women who are always desperate to talk about emotions and never people who fall hard. While this is certainly not true, each person must have a certain level of emotional intelligence in a relationship. An ideal man is emotionally intelligent and is capable of dealing with a partner there. Women are better than men to take into account their partner's opinions and views, which is essential for a healthy relationship.

12. An ideal man respects your opinions and listens to what you have to say:

Being closed-minded is not a trait that is exclusive to a particular gender, but it is not a good sign if a man is convinced that he is always right and that he will never consider his argument. An ideal man values and listens carefully to your thoughts

13. An ideal man will celebrate your accomplishments:

It's vital to have a partner to honor your achievements to make you feel incredible but also too happy with their relationships than those who reacted negatively or were indifferent. An ideal man will appreciate your achievements and help you do properly.

14. An ideal man will share your values:

Having a common outlook in life might be key to a successful relationship, an ideal man would share your values and try to make his personality according to your values, and you are to solve our problems in the same way.

If your priorities are the same, you and your partner will share similar approaches to everything from socializing to work, and this will likely lead to a higher level of mutual respect.

15. An ideal man makes you feel relaxed:

Around him, you don't have to be' on.' You can only be yourself. You are confident weeping in front of him, shouting in front of him, and enjoying moments of silence. The good, the bad, the hung-over, he's seen, and he still loves you.

16. He's making you happy:

He's making you smile more than you frown. You're always excited when you're with him. He treats you like a queen, and he does his utmost to make you happy.

17. You're attracted to him.

You're attracted to him beyond that. Sometimes you look at him, and you think, "It may not be everybody's cup of tea, but it's beautiful to me."

18. He's loyal:

Your man should be faithful, and 400 percent committed to you. He has eyes only for you. You never have to worry about being unfaithful to him because he's all yours.

19. He's a good listener:

The man you committed should listen to you, and I mean, listen to you.

20. An ideal man is sensitive and romantic:

A patient guy is a caretaker. He shows you that by doing things, he's considerate just to put a smile on your face. He knows what counts are the little things. He does whatever he is able to do to make you feel special.

21. He's sweet:

He's kind and compassionate because he's taking care of you and your feelings. He's affectionate for not being able to help himself. In private, he's sweet to you, and also in public, of course. He can't wait every morning and night to kiss you.

22. He appreciates you:

He tells you that you look beautiful out of the blue. He raves about you to his mates because he knows that you are unique. He knows he's lucky in his life, and he's never letting you forget it.

23. He blends in with your life:

He spends time with his family, and you feel comfortable with his family. He makes an effort to be involved and includes the people you love in your life. He cares for and wants your friends to like him. He fits perfectly in your life.

24. An ideal man is willing to do anything for you:

He knows it's going to make you happy. He is planning things he knows you're going to enjoy. Since he loves you, he is willing to do anything for you.

Qualities of an ideal man:

If you're looking for the ideal man, here's a list of five essential qualities he's got to have. If you are an applicant who wants to become an ideal man, the following characteristics should be cultivated:

Character:

This is the main attribute needed to make another person happy. Beware! Integrity and authenticity are absent in a man's nature; then, he lacks all that a relationship needs to thrive.

Maturity:

Immature people like to show off; they hate commitment, they are uncertain about their future, and they are naive. For a woman, there is nothing worse than having to submit to an insecure man. A woman needs a strong and stable man by her side, one who knows where he's going in life, one who's courageous enough to solve problems with his own hands and can look after her as any right partner would.

Smartness:

Intelligent men think before they act or say anything. It helps them to think about the consequences, a quality that gives women around them extra love, trust, and confidence. With so many women throwing themselves out there at married men, this is, by far, a crucial quality in ensuring fidelity.

Compatibility:

This is the attribute that allows a man and a woman to work together well, like pieces of the puzzle.

Fear of God:

The man who fears God, especially when she is not around, will never betray his partner.

Confident:

The ideal man is very sure of what he has and can do with his abilities. He's the kind of man in any situation who sees the positive, even if there are clear signs to the contrary. The optimism is contagious, and all around him know the faith of hopelessness. And he's not the sort in marriage to be distracted by the success of a woman because he knows his position and importance.

Appearance freak:

Usually, the ideal man looks beyond what his eyes can see when he sets out or gets married. Instead of a pretty face and body, he's searching for a personality that can suit his own because he knows those things don't matter. A guy who, before a good character, finds physical beauty has a lot to grow up to do.

Principled and straightforward:

If he's saying its blue, then it's blue, and if he's saying its black, it's black. A person of his words is the ideal man. He has values that he works by and is continually trying to maintain. He is trustworthy, and for anything, he can't deceive a friend. He sticks with one woman when he dates. He's not the guy to run around.

Romantic and caring:

He is the ideal man if he remembers your birthday and anniversary and knows how to leave lovely notes and surprise gifts for you. An ideal man can balance his job and his commitment. He always cares about his girlfriend and would never miss an opportunity to let her know how much he loves her. Any man who is unable to spoil his wife is wrong.

Better person:

Having someone to share your life with and learn a lot from them is the primary reason for commitment. When you're in a relationship that lacks this primary benefit, then on the wrong person, it's just a waste of time. You're sure to be better with the ideal man with every day or moment that passes because he would ensure it. He will inspire you, support you, and make the best of you.

Chapter 2

What did it Mean to be in Love?

Loving someone means that you only have to worry about how he makes you feel loved, unusual or appreciated. Being in love means you're always thinking about how to make him feel loved because that's just as important to you.

Difference between loving someone and being in love?

It is essential to find out first if you love or are in love with the person after you can continue your relationship or help you with the potential commitment. It is difficult to tell the difference between loving someone and being in love with them, mainly if love is something new to you. Loving someone can feel as intense, emotional, and consuming as being in love, but it's different in the end. If you hold out in your love life for magic and butterflies, it is essential to recognize the main differences. If you are ever broken up with someone you thought was The One, you're probably going to be able to relate to this list. Here is the difference between loving someone and being in love with them.

1. Loving Is a Choice, In Love Isn't:

You can choose someone to love. You can want to see their best qualities, respect them for who they are, and be their partner in helping them. You can also choose to stop loving, walking away, and forgetting about someone. It's not a choice to be in love. It's something that can happen without your intention or permission, so you can't walk away from it. You will take the feeling of being in love with you if you leave.

2. To love someone means to do them well, to be in love means to put the first:

Of course, you want the person you like to do well, but are you prepared to make the required sacrifices to make that happen? You put the needs of each other first when you are in love because your happiness is related to theirs. Perhaps while you're studying, he's chipping in a little extra for rent, or maybe you're taking extra morning walk shifts with the dog because he likes to sleep in. If you put the needs of each other first, you achieve more than when each of you fends for yourself.

3. Loving someone is temporary, always being in love:

Love at any moment will end. He can do annoying things, or you get into a bad fight or your kind of in a funk. You no longer love him. It's not that fickle to be in love. It remains through the struggles, the lulls, and the full-blown crisis of existence. When the honeymoon phase is over, and life is a little more reasonable, only a good one will be the one where you are in love. You don't need constant excitement because, without it, your feelings are null.

4. Loving Some Means Needing the Around, being in Love Means Needing Them to Be Where They Are Happy:

You always want them to be around when you love someone. You're looking forward to them. More than anything, you want him to be with you. You want them to have a happy, balanced life when you're in love, which sometimes means spending time away from you. You want them to have time out with the girls, or time alone, or time without you to try a few hobbies. Feeling content is not always the same as being together.

5. Loving Someone Is a Rush, being in Love Is Steady Stream of Emotions:

Love someone may be the best, but it comes with low lows as well. Being in love is a steadier stream of joy, but in the long run, it is total happiness. The caring person's roller coaster can never last, and bad lows can be devastating. That's why so many people mistake loving to be in love, but the real deal will never make you feel like you're crashing and burning.

6. Loving Someone Is About How They Make You Feel, being in Love Is About How They Feel:

An ordinary response people give when asked why they love someone is, "Because of how they make me feel." That's a valid answer, but if it's all about how you feel, you're probably not in love. Loving someone means that you only have to worry about how he makes you feel loved, unusual, or appreciated. Being in love means you're always thinking about how to make him feel loved because it's just as important to you.

7. Loving Is Ownership, being in Love Is a Partnership:

You want them to be yours when you love someone. It's essential to label them. You need them to be your boyfriend and tell them to be yours. It's about wanting to be in love with each other. You're giving up as much as you will. You two are a partnership, a team, to which no one belongs.

8. Loving is a battle of uphill; being in love is without effort:

You'll hear people say, "It's not supposed to be that hard." And they're right; it's not supposed to be. It's not in love to fight and scrabble to stay connected to keep the fire alive. You may love this person, but it inevitably turns into a situation in which you feel you're just forcing him. I'm not saying it's always going to be easy to have a relationship with someone you're in love with, just that the feeling of being in love without any effort. It's going to be trying some days. It seems to take all you have for a few days. But you'll always feel like you're in love with each other at the end of the hard days, or the hard months. That feeling is never going to be a job or effort.

How to Know That You Are in Love?

Knowing that you are in love with everyone feels different. Others have often been in love and are well acquainted with the emotion, and others may not be so sure if it is love or a deep infatuation.

Luckily, your body has pretty sneaky ways to tap you off to see if these emotions are more than just a passing phase for your mate. The next time you find yourself asking if you're actually in love, keep an eye out for these tell-tale signs.

If your partner has ever caught you lovingly staring at them, it could be a sign that you're heading over heels. Eye contact means you're fixed on something, so you might fall in love if you notice your eyes fixed on your friend.

When you're in love, what happened to your body and brain?

Your cheeks flush when you fall in love, your heart beats faster, your palms are sweaty, and your head begins to spin. All of this is due to a rush of chemicals and hormones flooding your brain and body when you fall in love. In this region, which is the same part of the brain involved in obsessive-compulsive behavior, leaves you with feelings of euphoria close to the "runner's high" endorphin-induced. During the attraction phase, blood flows to the pleasure center of the brain when you feel an overwhelming attachment to our partner

Research has also found that couples who lock eyes report feeling a romantic connection stronger than those that do not. It also goes the other way: they expressed romantic feelings to each other when a study saw strangers locking eyes for minutes at a time.

You Feel Like You Are High:

If you fall for someone, it's normal to feel out of your mind.

A Kinsey Institute study found that a person's brain that falls in love looks the same as a person's brain that takes cocaine. You should thank you for the feeling of dopamine, which is released in both situations.

This is a clear explanation for why people in new relationships are going to behave absolutely nonsensically.

You might feel you can't get them out of your brain if you love someone. This is because when you fall in love with someone, your brain releases phenyl ethylamine, called the "love drug." This hormone produces your partner's sensation of infatuation.

You may be familiar with the feeling as chocolate often includes phenyl ethylamine, which may explain why, after only one square, you can't stop.

You Want Them to Be Happy:

Love is an equal partnership, but when you fall for them, you will find that the happiness of someone becomes very important to you.

According to research, so-called "compassionate love" maybe one of the most excellent signs of a healthy relationship. This means you're willing to go out of your way to make life easier and happier for your partner.

> When you find yourself going out of your way to keep your companion safe as you walk in the rain or breakfast them on a busy weekday morning, it's a bad sign.

Even though love is often synonymous with warm and fuzzy feelings, it can also be an immense source of stress. Being in love also causes the stress hormone cortisol to be released from your brain, which can make you feel the sun.

So if you've noticed that your patience is being tested a bit more than usual or you're freaking out, you might not have to carry a stress ball yet; you might be in love.

You wouldn't experience pain as highly:

It might be traumatic to fall for someone, but if you found that falling doesn't bother you anymore., it might be a big sign that you're in love.

You Are Trying New Things:

Everyone at the beginning of their relationships wants to impress their date, but if you are always trying new things that your partner loves, you might have been bitten by the bug of love.

Nonetheless, a study found that after commitment, people who claimed to be in love often had different interests and personality traits. Like even if you dislike your partner's square-dancing class, it could have a positive impact on your personality.

Your Heart Rate Synchronizes with Theirs:

If you think about the one you love, your heart may skip a beat, but a study has shown that you may also beat each other in time. Research suggests that the souls of couples begin to beat at the same rate when they fall in love.

You might not be able to tell if this has happened without a couple of stethoscopes, feeling a deep connection with your partner is a good sign that you are in love.

You're OK with the Gross Stuff:

You might be in love if you're a notorious germaphobe and completely cool kissing your partner. Yes, a study found that feelings of sexual excitement can outweigh feelings of being grossed out.

So if you're attracted to your partner, that means you can just let them dip twice. It's love, honey.

You Get Sweatier:

You either have a terrible stomach bug or fall in love if you're nauseous and sweaty. A study found that falling in love, like sweat, can cause you to feel sick and display physical symptoms similar to anxiety or stress.

While this feeling is likely to pass once you're comfortable with your partner, it might be a good idea to carry an extra hanky to be safe.

You Love Their Quirks:

If you get to know a person, you're likely to pick things that make them unique. And if you're in love with them, they're probably some of the things you're most attracted to.

A study found that, as people have specific tastes, small differences can make a person love someone deeper than just physical appearance. At first glance, you may have judged your partner a bit harshly, if you notice that you are unexpectedly in awe of their uniqueness, you may be in love.

What's The Sense of Falling in Love?

To fall in love means you have someone on your side at all times. For better or worse, falling in love feels like pressing the restart button. It's like you forget what it feels like, or at least don't care to get hurt.

If you're in love, you start to think that your beloved is unique. The assumption is synonymous with an inability to feel anybody else's romantic desire.

Focusing On the Positive:

People who are genuinely in love tend to focus on their beloved's positive qualities while overlooking their negative characteristics. We also dwell on trivial things and items that remind them of their loved one, dreaming of these precious moments and memories day after day. However, in the presence of new stimuli, this is due to high rates of central dopamine and a jump in central norepinephrine, a chemical associated with increased memory

As is well known, falling in love also leads to physiological and psychological instability. You bounce between excitement, euphoria, increased energy, sleeplessness, and loss of appetite, trembling, a racing heart, accelerated breathing, anxiety, panic, and feelings of desperation when your relationship suffers even the smallest setback. These mood swings correlate to drug addicts' behavior. And indeed, when images of their loved ones are shown to in-love people, it fires up the same brain regions that trigger when a drug addict takes a hit. Researchers say that being in love is a form of addiction.

Intensifying Attraction:

We tend to intensify romantic attraction by going through some adversity with another person. Central dopamine may also be responsible for this reaction, as research shows that when a reward is delayed, neurons generating dopamine become more active in the mid-brain region.

Intrusive Thinking:

People in love report that, according to Fisher, they spend more than 85% of their waking hours musing over their "love object." It may result from reduced levels of core serotonin in the brain, a disorder typically associated with obsessive behavior, as this type of obsessive behavior is called intrusive thought.

Emotional Dependence:

People in love often display signs of emotional dependency on their relationship, including possessiveness, envy, fear of rejection, and anxiety about separation. For example, Fisher and her peers stared at the minds of people watching the pictures of a refused loved one or someone they were still in love with after getting rejected. "Activating areas involved in cocaine addiction may help to explain the obsessive behaviors associated with love rejection,"

Planning a Future:

They are also looking for emotional union with their beloved, seeking ways to get closer and dreaming together about their future.

"Functional MRI research shows that primitive neural systems underlying drive, reward recognition, and euphoria are active in nearly everybody when looking at their beloved's face and thinking loving thoughts. It positions romantic love in the company of mechanisms of survival, like those that make us hungry or thirsty, "I think of romantic love as part of a human reproductive strategy. It allows us to form pair-bonds that allow us to thrive. We have been created to experience the magic of love and be motivated toward others."

Compassion:

People who are in love feel a strong sense of empathy for their loved ones, feel the pain of others as their own, and are willing to sacrifice something.

Possessive Feelings:

Those who are genuinely in love usually experience sexual desire for their loved one, however strong emotional strings are attached: the desire for sex is combined with possessiveness, a passion for sexual exclusivity, and intense jealousy when the partner is accused of infidelity. Such possessiveness is believed to have developed so that an in-love person compels her spouse to spurn other suitors, thereby ensuring that the courtship of the couple is not disrupted until conception has taken place.

Chapter 3

Life Changes

How loves affect a personal life?

We are all evolving from those we were the year before into diffcrent people. We are changing our tastes, developing and expanding our skills, facing challenges that will help us in new and better ways. The things that we experience every day affect us in ways that we can see immediately and see later down the road, making every day our journey through life truly meaningful. Just like anyone else who walks the Earth, when you are in love your life also changed, as a result of a new feeling or the introduction of a new person into your life, we all experience these moments in life, an event in your life that has changed you in different ways than you could ever imagine. You have fallen in love with an incredible man, your life is that and changing for the better because of it.

First of all, you begin to be the best person you can be. It starts that way because you want to see your new love at your best: being a kind, smart, compassionate, and generally lovable guy. You want to make your partner happy and make them fall in love with you even more than they are because you love them so much and never want to end it. Eventually, however, you'll find that you're not the best person you can be because it's fun to see, but instead, your partner can help bring the attributes out of you. You don't try to be that awesome person because you've become that individual. You and the one you love can easily allow these incredible qualities to shine, and you realize that because of the one you like, you are ultimately a better person.

You're not only becoming a more powerful version of yourself, but you're also gaining skills you've never learned in life. Skills like knowing how to rub a certain way back, knowing what to say to make the one you love feel better, or picking the perfect place to eat that day. You'll learn how to fold your clothes in a certain way, what to make them after a rough day for dinner, how to play your favorite video game, and how to drive your car. You become a style expert, a food critic, a caretaker, a therapist, and a giver of warmth, and you get to learn these skills very quickly. Loving someone means learning new skills; you conclude that they are pretty good skills to have throughout your life.

You develop your pair of shorthand's once you've been together for a while. This particular language of yours allows communicational access for both of you with the bonus of confusing the hell out of everybody else around you. Perhaps the communication is made up of certain facial expressions or signals of the body. Maybe you two should interact by various pitched sounds that you can convey your feelings or thoughts. Perhaps you're using one-word responses that give you two more details than an explanation article. The two of you have a code, no matter what it is, and only other people wanted to communicate like you.

Love keeps growing, you find simple tasks quite fun, as you have someone to do with them all of a sudden. Washing your car becomes a challenge where you can clean your hand as quickly as possible. Shopping at the grocery store becomes a stupid banter or a race through the store.

With the changes in taste that you have in your life, you find that you are unexpectedly beginning to enjoy many of their feelings and vice versa. You're trading music from different artists back and forth; you're playing various types of games and discovering you're good at some of them, you're trying new things in life because they're interested in something and you're trying it out. These new tastes help bring you closer together, and you enjoy everything they do for both of you and the new doors that they open in your life. Maybe at a concert put on by one of their favorite bands, you'll share a life-changing moment. Or perhaps you're going to fall in love with a new recipe because your food choices have been changed. Maybe you're going to make a fantastic memory because you've been to a place they love and you've never been to. There are endless possibilities. All you have to do is try something new. There's no end of all the things you gain that change in your love. You've got your man's devotion. Your life has changed in incredible ways.

How love changes you?

When you think about how you feel like being in love, you start smiling. The smile is for the enlightening feeling when you first fall in love.

There are different kinds of love? Yeah, but every time you change yourself in some way or another love. This makes you in the present who you are. Your life and lost love encounters and struggles make you special individuals.

Love changes you:

It can do good things for your life, or it can take you down the wrong path. Anyway, love has this crazy impact on you. It maybe takes you to some very dark places in our lives, but it can also lead you on an even better path. It's always been this overwhelming feeling of happiness and freedom when you fell in love. The sense of freedom is in the person, and life's potential comes from love. You feel like you can do something and want to work harder on your goals and dreams, not just for yourself, but now for others that are important to you. That's what it should be like. Think back to the first time you've fallen in love with someone head over heels. Think back to that moment when either you wanted to concentrate on them, or you wanted to do great things with your life. You see, it can be good as well as evil.

The good, the poor, and the ugly:

Let's start with the ugly and the bad. There are types of love that will just destroy you if you're not in a good place in your life. There are people out there who only make you fall in love with them to benefit from you and your feelings. It's bad. Love makes you do stupid things in many of these situations. Only think of the consequences: you end up pushing loved ones away, you end up not thinking about your interests, your self-esteem usually goes down a long way, and you tend to do things that benefit the other person only. To encourage yourself to succeed, it's a pretty low and dark place.

And then the value is there. The love that you feel is amazing, uplifting, inspiring, and satisfying. Oh, what a happy feeling it is to be in love at the right time with the right person. Because it's all timing, so many wonderful perks come with the good about being in love. My preference is motivation. Just as it's said, we should all inspire and elevate each other, in a partnership the same goes. When you meet someone that makes you want to do better in all aspects of your life, well, it's just a feeling of joy.

Imagine going through life, working towards your goals and dreams, working hard in your career, and coming home every day knowing that your significant others are there to support you and just want you to be the best you can be. Whether or not having the support of the person you love speaks wonders about the person with whom you are. So when you're with someone who makes you feel happy and loved, happiness comes out of your aura.

Next, you always want to do something for yourself, not in an egoistic manner. More like it should be for yourself and then for your significant other to work towards your dreams and goals. Love, you see, does not completely change you, but in a way that awakens our souls and fills our hearts with joy. When it comes to you, it's a good thing to embrace.

You find yourself trying to find the right words if you try to explain love to people who haven't witnessed it. But to explain love, you usually find one or two precise words. In the end, when love changes you because it can and will choose the right path and know the right kind of love is the right path. Embrace it straight at full speed and consider who you are on the way there. Let love not describe you, but let it shine through you.

How love affects your physical health?

Love and affection for that particular person in your life have so many effects on our health. This leads to both short-term and long-term satisfaction and can enhance physical, psychological, and mental health through euphoric feelings and power of love.

It can improve physical, emotional, and mental health with the euphoric feelings and power of love.

Physically Love Affects Us Can Bring Us a Physical Reaction:

A fast-paced heart rate, butterflies in our stomachs, dilated pupils, sweaty palms, hard to find words, the instinctive urge to touch physically are just a few ways that love can affect us materially.

Sex will reap many benefits as a physical act of love. It can reduce blood pressure, increase women's bladder control, reduce stress, improve sleep, and boost the immune system. Such positive physical, sexual results will spill into many other aspects of life, from parenting to working to relationships and beyond.

A stable and healthy physical relationship often improves emotional and mental well-being with another person.

Love Promotes Emotional and Mental Wellbeing:

Several studies have shown that a good, supportive relationship, whether romantic, family, friendship, or otherwise, can be associated with higher self-esteem, increased self-worth, and increased self-confidence. Loving helps people integrate healthier habits into their daily lives, reduces anxiety (worry, nervousness), And decreases the likelihood of developing depression or other forms of mental illness, regardless of how it occurs.

Love Changes Your Brain Chemistry:

Love momentarily changes your brain chemistry. You will relate the brain chemicals to those butterflies that flutter in your belly. It can also be correlated with releasing brain chemicals to your heart's thrilling feeling of missing a beat or leaping out of your brain. Romance can be linked to several brain chemicals and hormones, but two stand out individually:

Dopamine and oxytocin.

Dopamine is basically a chemical in the brain that releases something pleasurable when you see or feel something. It's making you want more of it. Dopamine is what can make love, and it seems irresistible to your significant other. It is the same chemical in the brain that perpetuates changes such as gambling, misuse of drugs, etc. You can feel like you're on a high when you meet a new particular person and want more and more of that person.

Oxytocin, a hormone that calms and helps bind partners, helps foster trust between two individuals. It is also called the "cuddle hormone," which is released when you play with or pet your dog.

Often these changes are only temporary in brain chemistry and hormones. Once the new particular individual becomes the new normal in your life, you must adapt back to standard brain chemistry.

Falling Out of Love Hurts:

If for one reason or another, someone you love hurts us or is no longer part of our lives, our health can hit us. The same pain receptors are used by physical and emotional emotions, and to feel those feelings; our brain uses the same neurological pathways.

You may have learned of broken heart syndrome, but you may not know it's a real medical disorder that can affect your physical, psychological, and mental health. Broken heart syndrome is also called stress-induced cardiomyopathy, where a serious and sometimes lethal condition is temporarily swelled by the chest. The disorder may occur during a break-up or divorce, mourning for a loved one who has been seriously injured or departed, or during a time of extreme stress.

Love:

While everyone has different experiences of love, everyone has the ability regardless of age, gender, sexual orientation, race, ethnicity, religion. Love comes in many different ways throughout your life and relationships and manifests in many different ways. After being profoundly hurt by someone you love or losing someone you love, healing, moving on to the next stage of your life, and finding happiness and love again may seem impossible.

You're likely to feel the fluttering butterflies in your stomach, clammy palms, and high dopamine that comes with experience finding new love, searching for the soul, self-discovery, and opening up to new experiences.

Chapter 4

What is Meant by Lifetime Commitment?

What Is Commitment?

Commitment involves engaging in something like a person or a cause. Think before you commit. An activity needs you to do something. Some commitments are significant, like marriage. Did you ever make a commitment to yourself or someone, and for whatever reason?

There are numerous definitions for the word "commitment," the most basic description being an "act of voluntarily assuming and fulfilling obligations," which is, in fact, further defined as "social" and not as a professional or organizational commitment. What makes it so personal is the voluntary nature of personal engagement. This does not mean, however, that an activity has to appeal only to individual interests, such as human relationships or core beliefs. With a personal commitment, mutual acceptance of all commitments, every target can be achieved. It is possible to devote any number of projects and causes, including an organization, a team, a religious group, or other entity.

Most successful people have commented on the fact that commitment is a significant factor in individual success. This is usually because the individual has to lead his or her cause for some time, at least until others can join the cause. For any plan to succeed, action must be taken first, and commitment is what motivates people to act. Commitment involves not only committing one's self to a purpose but also regularly practicing this belief system. It would be misleading to describe commitment as persistence alone; it is persistence with intent or aim and based on a reasoning basis that is closely linked to the core beliefs of an individual (or group).

Some of the most successful entrepreneurs in modern times are individuals who have been described as "committed" to their profession or cause, as well as throughout history. Usually, they are not people of extraordinary genius, nor have they built an empire based on blind luck. We are people who have firmly adhered to a set of obligations and have seen them through.

What does it mean to you?

In this life, each of us has the destiny to fulfil. In this lifetime, each of us has a target. If you've got to do some more essential things in your lifetime, it doesn't mean you're luckier or more important than anybody else. It's just because each of us has an individual soul that comes with our universe's consciousness and awareness. There's a place for your heart. So you've got a mission. The truth is that your soul is here for your life experiences and lessons to evolve.

In the first place, therefore, we all have a dedication to our hearts, and it should not be seen as unusual for us to revisit and assess this commitment from time to time. It's essential for you not to lose track of where you are heading in our lives as far as our intent or destiny is concerned; otherwise, it's going to be a waste of existence.

Commitment can be described with yourself in this context as honest and sincere. It is your goal to fulfil the promise you made to your soul when you understand your personality and are present in today's life. That's the self's dedication.

This is a strict commitment to accept in the first place and, in reality, the judgment you await when you pass over when the soul itself makes our physical life ends based on what has been accomplished with that life's experiences. As many of you claim, it is not God who judges you!

Some people may be puzzled about this and wonder, "How can you ever pledge to a person you've never seen or heard of before you've even been born? "Well, after previous unfulfilled commitments and the inability to fulfil our destiny on this planet in a lifetime, that commitment was overdue. Souls continue to come after lifetime for human experiences only to satisfy unfulfilled chances of a previous life. Don't you think what a waste of a ride here? For most of us, the main reasons for failure are straightforward. The causes are due to our limited vision of life, our lack of understanding of our world, and eventually our shortcomings depending on the system of belief or faith to which we belong or the community with which we evolve or the environment to which we are accustomed.

Commitment Starts with You First:

I have a responsibility to myself, and at the same time, everyone should be committed to themselves. What does self-commitment mean to you? Is that in your own life for you?

Usually, you start dating another person when it comes to relationships with others. On many occasions, you are not even prepared to make any commitment to anyone else. It may also take a couple of shots in a relationship before you wake up and realize you must first commit to yourselves. Why do you have to commit to your life to be with someone else? Is it for safety? Or is that dependence? Or is it just anxiety to be alone?

We produced a marriage ritual on this flight. Marriage is like a protective umbrella that we use to describe and classify as committed. We recite in front of a judge, a priest, a rabbi, or whatever authority we identify with our promise of commitment to each other. That's all very good, but remember, the truth these days is that more and more divorces are going on around us and the world. Okay, in this situation, it must mean that our plan to commit ourselves to another person is something very wrong. Either that or we don't grasp our commitment's obligation. One possible explanation for this is, among other reasons, our lack of commitment to ourselves.

If two people decide to get committed, they place their engagement in front of each other on the table, as well as their family and friends. If they can go that far, they should at least have a real awareness and understanding of the responsibility for what they get into. Before that pledge, we discussed being truthful with ourselves and being genuine. It is still important to be honest and correct with the other person when it comes to two people and to respect your loyalty to the soul of each other. It also means that when you say all this, no one will manipulate the other because that's not what commitment is about. No one is going to derail the other from completing their dedication to their hearts. Alternatively, two people should share and be transparent and nourish the interest of each other. You don't have precisely the same fate.

Why commitment is important in life?

A commitment is a decision that needs you to take a certain course of action. Whatever the topic, whether it's a healthy existence, a better relationship, or a refreshed approach to work commitment, is one of the most important principles for success.

What is meant by lifetime commitment?

Lifetime Commitment is about sharing, respecting, growing, and prospering with the commitment of each other without either of you being involved in controlling, manipulating, invading, or abusing the other in any way.

Commitment Is Essential for a Long-term Relationship

Real, long-term relationships are built on much more than compatibility and chemistry. Commitment is the key ingredient that keeps everything together.

Commitment acts as the assurance of a promise, a guarantee you made the personal agreement with the one you love. It's not just about maintaining your duty during days of fair weather. No. Commitment comes into play much more when it comes to hurricanes. This shows in your resolve to respect your duty by remaining thick and thin with each other.

It is so necessary, for those very reasons, to remind your partner of your daily dedication. You will need to express it with honesty to do that.

Commitment in Relationships

Emotional relationships are very significant, including family relationships, friendships, and romantic relationships. All of them are based on love, but what is involved in love? How critical in relationship commitment is?

The three most important aspects of any relationship are love, confidence, and dedication. We're going to discuss the communication.

We need to know what it is and be able to distinguish it from the other two things before we start to examine whether participation in relationships is advantageous or not.

What does commitment mean?

Commitment is the willingness of people to stay together. All partnerships require some degree of responsibility. Family or friendship is different from a romantic partner's commitment. Romantic relationships generally require more engagement than bonds.

Commitment in simple terms is a type of social contract that is accepted by both parties. It is what seals the deal that you label yourself as "friends," "a couple," or "married." The problem is that each party usually does not explicitly outline the specific clauses of this contract. The content of that contract tends to reflect the expectations that society believes that each party should meet.

The main objective of engagement in relationships is to feel a sense of security and control for each party. You feel comfortable with certain expectations about how your partner should behave when you're in a contract. This lets you anticipate the types of situations that may occur and act accordingly.

It is useful in many respects to have some leverage and feel secure in relationships. For example, when a couple is dedicated to each other, raising children becomes easier. This is because children are born wholly defenceless, and they need constant care of their parents.

So what does this mean nowadays? People generally agree that marriage requires a few things: loyalty: many people consider cheating a strong reason for ending a romantic relationship.

A willingness to keep the relationship going for the foreseeable future: if one of the partners wants to break up after a short period of time, you should probably agree that they have not been committed.

Is the commitment a good thing or a bad thing?

When you pay close attention to your relationships, you will see that, to some degree, many of them are toxic. This is because relationship engagement can lead to many problems because of: the implicit social contract.

This carries with it the hopes.

Implicit social contract:

Implicit social contracts are the terms that must be fulfilled by each partner. The spouses do not express what they want from each other in most situations.

On the contrary, with certain expectations about how their partner should behave, they start their relationship.

Each individual has its interpretation of the implications of engagement in relationships. Thus, due to these individual expectations, many conflicts may arise at the beginning of the relationship.

Social expectations:

When you're engaged to another individual, you've got a set of ideas on how to make your partner happy. Problems arise, however, when one partner does not meet the expectations of the other.

Overall, both parents try to meet the expectations of the other. Sometimes, though, they do this by compromising their own needs. This may eventually lead to unhappiness.

The need for control:

Eventually, the need to control our partner will make you feel committed. This may be embedded in your protection need. The problem is that power can lead to dependence on emotion. Eventually, your partner may feel trapped and frustrated as such.

Autonomy is a need for a man. We cannot pressure others to act following our laws. A subordination-based relationship impedes freedom. And this leads to unhappiness and disappointment.

Rational vs. Emotional Commitment:

Rational vs. emotional engagement is quite let and touches on the conversation we had during lunch. You might wonder about the difference between rational and emotional engagement.

Rational engagement is the one you agree to give your time, talent, and resources to an organization in return for financial compensation, incentives for professional development, and the ability to achieve your career ambitions.

The passion and intent behind the work is emotional commitment. What keeps you in the organization's relationship?

As you enjoy your trust increases when you are emotionally committed, and your heart flutters with complete satisfaction.

Rationally dedicated workers do what they need to do; emotionally committed staff do what they want to do.

Although this in itself is pretty cool, it goes further. Recently, the Corporate Leadership Council surveyed 50,000 employees from 59 different organizations in 27 countries, representing ten industry groups. Emotional connection is 4 times as necessary to drive discretionary effort as rational commitment among employees.

Discretionary effort means raising your hand to take on more jobs, offering to help someone when they are overwhelmed, and proactively walking the extra mile to achieve results without anyone hitting you on the shoulder to ask for your help.

Your brilliance is ignited when you're emotionally committed to your organization because you're not wondering if you're valued and safe in your position.

What does it mean to committed to someone?

Commitment is not just about being able to sit still with your partner and keep your eyes closed. It's not just about avoiding the world's temptations. It's not just about saying no to all the possibilities of unfaithfulness and infidelity. Commitment is so much more than simply choosing to go home every night to a single person. Commitment is not only a physical connection between two individuals. Commitment is the establishment with another person of an exclusive emotional connection.

You don't feel the need to have any of those dating apps on your smartphone when you commit to someone because you know you don't need an app to find the love of your life. You've already seen that one person who's stolen your heart. You're always satisfied with that person when you commit to someone, and you wouldn't even entertain the idea of being a two-timer. Once you engage in a relationship, you lose any opportunities to engage in a relationship with other people. That's what it should feel like for real commitment, and that's what it is.

When you really commit to someone, you give up all your days of being flirtatious with other people. Romance and love are no longer a challenge for you. You no longer see love and romance as a challenge, you have to win because by finding your soul mate, you have already won. If you are loyal to someone, you must automatically shut down any advances made by any third party on you. You're wearing the engagement tag on your neck mechanically by saying you're taken, and you're off the market. You don't want to entertain someone new because this one particular person has already taken up all the space in your mind. When you're in a genuine, committed relationship with someone, then outside the link, you're not taking part in any foolish monkey business. For the hell of it, you don't want to lead other people on. You don't feel the need to attract other people to you because your partner's attraction is always more than sufficient.

Practicing real commitment means you will never hide from other people your relationship status. You're proud to wear it around your neck like a medal to see the whole world. You never want to give the idea to others that your relationship is rocky or that you can steal. You are not at your disposal. You're being taken, and you're proud of that. You are finally off the market, and you want to put it to the world's attention. You don't need all those little confidence boosters from outside sources because it's more than enough to raise the trust you get from your partner. You're committed to your partner's idea and nobody else. That's what a real commitment is. If you choose to commit to someone, you're almost giving up a considerable amount of your privacy and individuality. This means you're willing to share with another person a big part of your life. It indicates that at all times, even when the truth hurts or inconveniences you, you must be committed to being honest with that person. Being dedicated to someone implies that at all hours of the day, you encourage yourself to be free. It means you should be receptive to anything that your partner might want or have to tell you. Being in a committed relationship ensures you have ample respect for each other to understand each other the truth at all times.

It's a challenging thing to be devoted to another human, but it's not entirely impossible. If you are genuinely committed to someone else, it means that you must continuously make an effort to learn more about the person with whom you are. Being committed means you're open to making the adjustments you need to make your partner happy, and being committed implies that for the sake of the relationship, you are willing to make some compromises here and there. You always work tirelessly continuously to make sure your connection remains smooth regardless of how hard it gets. That's what it feels like for real dedication. You never get tired of putting each other at work.

Ultimately, being involved in a relationship means being able to trust the independence of one another. You have to commit yourself and your connection to the idea. If you want to commit to each other, you have to be able to respect the autonomy of each other. Commitment isn't something right off the bat that can be flawless. It has to be built. It's got to work on it. But all partnerships will always survive on mere participation at the end of the day.

5 Ways You Can Communicate Your Commitment to Your Spouse or Long-Term Partner:

Communication includes expressions, both verbal and nonverbal. While it is important to say something with words, it is more convincing to demonstrate it with corresponding acts. Therefore, consider using these five basic and concrete ways to communicate to your partner your devotion.

1. Show love and loyalty:

Loving means, saying to your mate, "I love you," including romantic gestures and sexual desire signals. Yet you will also have a strong desire to show your commitment to your partner's well-being and satisfaction.

You should be your spouse or partner with whom you want to spend your time. The company's ambition should be clear.

By always speaking positively about your relationship, you will show your love and devotion while keeping in touch with your partner.

2. You can only express this sincerely when you feel respect and appreciation for your partner:

Appreciation and appreciation for kind contact will allow you to show your love for your partner. Supporting and encouraging their feelings will help them feel like they can always seek advice and comfort from you.

Take the time to hear your mate truly. Also, don't be afraid to share your own emotions. Be polite, use respectful words, and try to get a deeper understanding of your mate. It will show the depth of your commitment to express your personal interest in them.

3. It is impossible to convey trust and honesty in a relationship without trust:

Therefore, the formation and transmission of trust call for complete honesty. Your partner can only have an accurate picture of who you really are when you commit to being honest.

Be frank with your past and be truthful with your future vision. Share your feelings, share your thoughts, and share with your mate your very presence. Do all you can to prevent lies or half-truths from undermining your faith and devotion?

4. Working as a team and compromise:

Teamwork shows commitment as it often calls for compromise in your willingness. This ensures that you are as worried about the needs of your partner as you are your own. You must stop being single-minded and shift your thinking from "mine" to "our" from "me" to "we." Show your partner appreciation and willingness to make concessions. You don't have to affect your individual moral values and standards adversely. Just be open to hearing the views, wishes, and dreams of your mate and don't impose on them. Keep your individuality, but work with each other.

5. Disagree agreeably:

Showing your partner's commitment doesn't mean you're never going to fight or disagree. You're two people. Conflict must occur. It's when you threaten just to throw it all down and leave that you undermine your relationship's commitment.

Therefore, be sensitive when conflict arises. Don't yell or hurl your partner's accusations that you will regret later. Instead, listen with curiosity and a desire for understanding to your mate. If everything else fails, agree to disagree with respect.

Remaining sensitive and supportive during difficult times is the best way to express commitment.

Tell yourself how hard it would be to enforce and express your commitment to these suggestions. If you really love your partner, you will feel like reasonable and normal steps to these five points. It's your choice to take them.

11 Signs that you are in a lifetime Commitment

So you want to know if it's a committed relationship. It is not enough these days to believe the conventional "boyfriend," "girlfriend," or even "partner" tags are adequate to affirm the status of exclusivity. In addition to the more obvious actions of living together and getting involved, there are some things that never change, and if your relationship has any of the following characteristics, there is a strong possibility that you will be in a committed one.

1) When two people spend a lot of time together.

One of the very first signs of engagement in a relationship is spending time together Outside of normal working hours; there is usually not much time left to spare with all the things you could do in a day. As of time is one of very few goods that no one can get back, it's a good sign that you're both committed to making time for each other regularly.

2) You involve each other in your daily purchases:

I had a friend who admitted to me that the day she found herself in the supermarket with more products in her cart for her partner than for herself, she realized that she was in a committed relationship and that they didn't even live together. Such thoughtful acts can be small and apparently insignificant or as extravagant as purchasing matching jewellery. Whatever the purchase, you are definitely in a committed relationship if you have each other in mind to the point where you are considering them in your regular purchases.

3) You get a Key:

Recall that it wasn't a big deal to give someone a key to your house.

If you have keys to the house of the other one or both of you, you're in! I mean, how many people have your place keys? There aren't many chances, but if they do and they aren't your family, it's a good sign that you're in a committed relationship.

4) You Don't Shun Social Media Shout-Outs:

In this era of media mayhem, it's no wonder that a public announcement on some form of social media appears to be one of the first signs of commitment. You've seen them: the sulfide of the infamous couple, the sweet message for everyone to see, and the hashtags like "me and my son." Such public displays are usually a pretty good sign that things are going well and that you're both confident enough to express your love to the world. These public displays can only mean "we have dedicated ourselves, and we want to meet everyone."

5) Entering into a major contract:

I think it's reasonable to say that somebody (like buying a home or a car), is a sign that it's fairly serious between you. The possible explanation why agreements are so big is that they're usually much simpler to get out of than they're going to get into, this is why most people are careful when signing on the piece of paper and expect long time to engage.

6) You Holiday Together:

Holidays usually take place over several days and can sometimes take several weeks, so if you're going to take company along, you're going to want to make sure that you really like them. You're also making life-long memories. Generally speaking, people who spend their holidays together not only enjoy the company of each other, but you're able to celebrate together, so if you spend your holidays together, it's a good sign that you're truly committed to your relationship.

7) You're talking about corporeal functions:

You certainly don't chat around the dinner table about your groin injury or irritable bowel syndrome. Normally, these talks are reserved for medical appointments and sometimes funny stories. Nonetheless, if you find that you can talk about intimate body functions with your partner, you are definitely more than casual friends, especially if you find that usually private and personal conversations are commonplace between you two.

8) You Plan for the Future Tog:

If you consider the average lifespan is between 70 or 80 years, you will spend one-third of that time asleep; it is significant that you and your sweetheart are talking about how to spend the hours you stay together. You can make decisions based solely on your wishes when you're single. However, what the other person wants to do and where they see themselves in the future is important in a committed relationship. So if you're planning together with your partner, there's a good chance your relationship will be in for the long haul.

9) You Share Passwords and PIN Numbers:

These days, with the limitations on the amount of personal privacy that any of us has, passwords and PIN numbers may mark the final boundary of the few things that we have full control over. So cannot be taken lightly or with casual friendships to decide to share this extremely private information. While experts admit that sharing passwords can reinforce relationships, this is a sign of commitment as it shows ultimate confidence. So, unless you're in a committed relationship, keeping your passwords and PIN numbers private is still the best practice.

10) You Go Out of Way for One Another:

Part of being a good citizen of the world is taking care of other people, which may sometimes involve going out of your way. But if it's less effort and more this-is - just-how-we-behave to go out of your way for your loved one, you've got yourself a keeper, and you're definitely committed. Examples of going out of your way may look like taking your lunch break to make an order for them, rearranging your travel plans to make sure they get the time off to be with you or giving up your car to make sure they do it on time (and vice versa, of course). Anything less is a committed one, and there is no assurance that you are a partnership.

11) You make decisions based on the situation of the other person:

Did your mate give up their favourite candy bar because of your nut allergy (no kissing for you) or traded in that beef-lover's pizza for your vegan? Well, you can be sure that there is no doubt that they are committed when they begin to make changes to their routines and behaviours based on your beliefs, situation, or circumstances.

Chapter 5

How to Find that He is Perfect for Your Lifetime Commitment?

The reasons you fall in love may be a mystery, but much less mysterious are the reasons we remain in love. There may be no such thing as the ideal partner but is someone who has developed in specific ways that go beyond the surface; an ideal partner can be found. Although we each pursue a different set of qualities that are specifically important to us individually, there are specific psychological characteristics that both you and your partner may seek to make the fire not only stronger, more intense and more satisfying but also far less likely to die out at midnight when the clock strikes.

Many of these qualities will not be apparent to us when we meet someone for the first time, but as we get to know the people we date, these are invaluable features to both looks in and strive for in ourselves. These attributes are ideal for

1. Maturity:

This statement is not intended to echo the ever-advised mantra of the importance of maturity. It's not just a matter of no longer behaving like a child to be "grown-up." It's not a boyfriend who avoids getting the trash out or a girlfriend who never runs late. These qualities are excellent, but to grow means making an active effort to recognize and resolve our past negative influences. Therefore, an ideal partner can focus on its past and is interested in understanding how old experiences shape new behaviours.

When people mature emotionally, on their current relationships, they are less likely to re-enact or project past experiences. They develop a strong sense of independence and autonomy, having distinguished themselves from early life from destructive influences. As they evolve within themselves, they are less likely to look for someone to compensate or complete their incompleteness for shortcomings and weaknesses. Instead, they are looking for someone to share their lives as equals and to appreciate themselves independently. This person is much more available to a romantic partner and the new family that they create together, having broken ties to old identities and patterns. Becoming emotionally mature helps us with this process and dramatically improves our chances of a stable and rewarding relationship.

2. Openness:

The ideal partner is an open, unprotected, and vulnerable partner. No human being is perfect, so it can be a tremendous asset to a lasting union to find someone who is accessible and receptive to feedback. When someone is free-thinking and open-minded, it allows them to be straightforward in expressing feelings, thoughts, dreams, and desires, letting you know them. Often, their transparency is an indicator of their engagement in personal development and often leads to the relationship's progress. Perfect relationships do not exist like perfect people, but finding someone you can talk to about an environment you believe is missing in your marriage and open to change is more than half the fight. By contrast, being willing to accept our partners ' feedback and seeking that kernel of truth in what they say allows us to develop similarly.

3. Integrity & Integrity

In a close relationship, the ideal partner recognizes the value of integrity. Honesty builds people's trust. The other person is confused by dishonesty, betraying their vulnerability and breaking their sense of reality. Nothing has a more destructive impact than fraud and deception on a close relationship between two people. The blatant deception involved is often equally, if not more, harmful than the unfaithful act itself, even in painful situations such as infidelity. The ideal partner aims to live a life of honesty so that words and actions do not differ. It extends to all contact levels, including verbal and nonverbal. In our most intimate relationships, being open and honest means understanding ourselves and our intentions. While it can be challenging to prove this, it is a worthwhile effort.

4. Respect & Independence:

Ideal partners appreciate the interests of each other separately from their own. They feel comfortable with each other's overall goals in life and support them. They are sensitive to the desires, desires, and feelings of the other and place them with their own on an equal footing. Of dignity and empathy, the best couples treat each other. With threatening or manipulative behaviour, they do not try to control each other. They respect the distinct personal boundaries of their partner while remaining physically and emotionally close at the same time. Valuing and respecting the sovereign minds of our partners and not trying to change them makes it possible for us to know them as individuals.

5. Empathy:

The ideal partner perceives both an intellectual level, an observational level, and an intuitive level of emotion. This person is capable of understanding and empathizing with his partner. As two people in a relationship understand each other, they are mindful of the commonalities between them, knowing and appreciating the differences as well. The growing partner feels recognized and respected when both partners are empathic, that is, able to communicate with feelings and appreciation for the interests, attitudes, and values of the other person. Developing our empathic capacity helps us understand and adapt to our mate.

6. Affection:

On many levels, the ideal partner is easily affectionate and responsive: physically, emotionally, and verbally. He or she is personal, recognizing and showing feelings of warmth and tenderness outwardly. In giving and accepting affection and pleasure, this person should enjoy closeness in being sexual and feel uninhibited. To be open to giving and receiving love adds to our lives a poignant feeling.

7. Humour:

The ideal partner is humorous. A sense of humour in a relationship can be a lifesaver. The ability to laugh at one's self and the weaknesses of life allows a person to maintain a correct perspective when dealing with sensitive issues arising within the relationship. Playful and joking partners, often with their laughter, defuse potentially volatile situations. A good sense of humour eases tense moments in a relationship. It makes life much easier to be able to laugh at ourselves. Moreover, being able to smile with someone close to us is one of the greatest joys of life.

He is fallen for you:

He doesn't tell you anything when you ask him if he loves you. Maybe he isn't the kind of person that talks too much. You want to be sure of your boyfriend as a woman. So you'd like to be sure of your choices. After all, with a dead-end relationship, no one wants to waste time or a guy who is not interested in giving everything. He loves you ten signs and sees if he has fallen for you in such a way that words cannot express his feelings.

1. He responds in no time:

You've only sent him, "Hey, sweetie, where are you?" And two seconds later, you received a reply with the full address and whereabouts of his place. He added, too, who he is with and when he returns. He then closes the text with a confirmation that he misses you that is always welcome. You're missing the point if you're still wondering how he can text it back so quickly. If it's not a sign he loves you, what is it then? The man is on fire with text messages, and there's something that tells me he can't take his eyes off his phone, continually checking if you've written him. Time is essential, and he can't wait until he gets your answer. You're here in something. The same applies to telephone calls.

2. He's doing it your way:

He complains about all the little things you're asking him to do now and then, yet he knows how essential they are, and he's going along with them. That must be a sign that he loves you! Let's face that. Women love being the boss at home. Some wives in the house can take this very seriously. So what's better than a man who leaves plenty of room to flow? There's no point in arguing anyway for small things. If you're searching for certain signs that he likes you, ask him on a Saturday night to go to a girly movie with you. If he says yes, it's because he's doing your way of doing things, and that's great.

3. He's treating you like a lady:

People, especially younger ones, haven't learned the right ways to treat a lady like you these days. You are lucky that your partner asked you, searched online, and found the secrets of treating you like a lady. Your boyfriend is more like a knight, a true gentleman who has grown up well. Your man is doing all a well-behaved person is doing to honour the lady next to him. He's always following you, for example, or walking next to you. He makes sure that when he's around, you never have to open a door. He never allows you to carry anything other than your bag. And even then, because he's more than happy to pay the bill, he never lets you use it. These are all clear signs that he loves you and that he values you as an individual, not because he is

4. He loves your natural beauty:

When you walk in the party, you might get a lot of heads to switch. You're an incredible princess who likes to impress. Yet he loves the way you pose with your pyjamas, even when you're dressed up. Even these days when you don't have any make-up and hate your frightened face. It's a sign that he loves you when he doesn't care about all the jewellery and phony stuff that you put on, but he respects you for who you are. Passion and desire are emotions that may attract men in the first place, but they hold them around with real love. And true love comes from real, natural beauty. Don't you ever forget that it will be very different in 10 years, no matter how amazing you might look at a typical Saturday out? So you need to have someone by your side who will look you 20 years down the road in your eyes and still be in love with you like he kissed you for the first time.

5. He doesn't want you to leave the bed if you don't have enough orgasms:

Most men don't care about the happiness of their bed mate. They want to satisfy their ego by conquering another lady. Your lover, however, ensures that you get the right attention in bed. He doesn't want to finish unless he makes sure you've had your life's time. So you still have fireworks in bed after two days, two weeks, or even two years. Research has shown that maintaining a healthy sexual relationship throughout the year is one of the most telling signs that he deeply loves you because he can't get enough of you.

6. When he's thinking to you, he's full of pride:

See him when he's speaking with his mates regarding you. If he's excited about explaining your new fitness success or how you got your promotion at work, then this must be one of the signs that he loves you. He admires your intellectual background, academic studies, or making more money than he does. The vast knowledge of world affairs and the great addition to the Friends TV show is something that scares him every day. To attract somebody's attention, you don't have to be a genius. One of the signs that he likes you is when the guy you are dating acknowledges that you succeed in every little thing, no matter how small it may be. He's fine with all that because he loves you deeply.

7. He is spoiling You:

He wakes up and goes straight to the kitchen for breakfast. Or he runs for delicious hot pastries to your favourite bistro. For your birthday, he buys the best gifts, and you always get something special for Christmas. The holiday season is around the corner, and he can't wait for you to go shopping. Or the other day, he booked tickets to Hawaii, making you your life's biggest surprise. He said when you asked why, because you deserve it. The fact that he pumps you even when there is no special occasion is one of the clearest signs that he loves you. Your husband is a part of the exclusive group of men more interested in you than his family. He's got his own life, but he's always putting you as a priority that you should be proud to feel and behave like that because it's not very normal!

8. He supports your dreams:

You may have crazy plans to be the next Top Model or to take over Oprah Winfrey when she retires. And to be the most famous pop star and sell millions of records. One of the signs that he loves you is that with your dreams, he never laughs, no matter how crazy they look. To help your choices, he's always behind you. Your boyfriend is going the extra mile to help you make your dreams come true. He deals with your goals as they were his. Not because he has no dreams of his own, but he wants to work with you. Your boyfriend feels it's a great way to get closer to you and show how much he cares for you. But plans have not always been as planned, and both of you know. Not an issue! One of the undeniable signs he loves you is that when you failed and realized how high you were setting the bar; he's got a tissue ready. He never says, "I've told you that." He'll be super supportive, on the contrary, and try to cheer you up, doing what you love best.

9. He doesn't mind behaving stupidly to make you laugh:

You've had the worst day of your existence, and he's just beginning to dance dangerously to cheer you up. One of the real signs that he loves you is that he does everything he needs to see you happy. No matter the cost, he'll do it if he'll put a smile on your face. Loving is not to take; it is to give. Your boyfriend knows deep inside him this universal truth, so at any given opportunity, he gives joy and happiness. It's because seeing you happy makes him feel satisfied when the man you're dating makes a real effort to see you smile. It's a sign that he's not been fruitless in his efforts to please you, that he manages to brighten your day. You can't help but accept these signs that he loves you, it's clear that he has strong feelings about you, you can't see

10. He listens carefully to you and follows your advice:

OK, let's face it. Maybe he'll never say you're right. But he's not the guy that's talking a lot anyway, remember? Look for signs that he loves you in actions in such cases, not words. It is more than enough to convince you that he respects your point of view that he takes your advice seriously and follows your recommendations. If your boyfriend is a great listener, you'll have to stick with him because you don't find guys like him. Most guys like talking all the time about themselves and being proud of what they're doing. These are not signs that he loves you, but rather indicates that he loves himself, in the universe more than anything else. And nobody likes to be with a big ego guy. Selfish people tend to think only on their own, and they never care. You also often have trust issues, and remaining in a long-term relationship without freaking out is going to be very difficult for them. When you think about it, it may be the last of the signs that he loves you!

You've Found Your Life Partner:

The desire to see our soul mates is almost impossible to escape: are there any signs that you have found your life partner I should look for?

It's more complicated than you might think, counsellor couples and marriage coach. "There's no' one' person, but more of a' perfect' type," "This type may change throughout your life because over the years we're not staying the same. Different qualities in your life may be relevant at different times. The one ' encompasses as many of these qualities as possible at one-time no one will fulfil them all. "Your one true love can contain multitudes and can affect your life in more ways than just one." The one "will not just smile on your face and give you butterflies; they will do that and much more.

1. He supports you:

Whatever the size of your dreams, "the one" will understand you and support you. They'll be right next to you, cheering you on, making your fifth pot of coffee, and rubbing your back when you need a rest when you're up for an exam all night long or trying to meet a work deadline.

"A valid measure of the quality of a relationship is to consider what it brings out in you and your life," "You are often happier and healthier when you are in healthy relationships."

2. He listens to you:

Whether it's about your mother or your best friend, "the one" is going to listen to you and hear every word.

"Everyone wants to be heard and understood, so it's also more important to be a good listener than to monopolize every conversation," online dating expert and award-winning dating coach, "Just say,' if they hear you and appreciate that you're sharing your thoughts and feelings with him,' will improve your communication skills."

3. He builds with you, not for you:

The two of you will work together as a team when you meet "the one." The essential quality in' one' is the commitment to work on it," "All the conditions mentioned above may exist when you're dating, but how do you continue to foster them in years? It's critical to find someone who wants that and wants to work with you. "It's going to build your future together, not separately.

4. You trust Him:

You'll know that when you can trust them entirely, you've found your guy.

"Trust provides the vital feelings of protection, security, and transparency for both dating partners and relationships experts say,' you can be more confident and deepen your bond and love. Without trust, a partnership will have a lot of negativity, depression, and disconnection.

5. Something you don't always have to do:

Not every day has to be packed with plans. Even the chilly days are magical when you're with your guy.

The one' includes a range of features such as compatibility, chemistry, deep love, appreciation, reverence, fun, and humour. Life will feel like an adventure from the minute you wake up, even if you're lying in bed.

6. He'll never put you down:

Your man will never let you feel "less than" because they'll be there to lift your trust and spirit.

"Healthy relationships have a nice balance to make us feel accepted and challenge us to grow," he will make sure you know you're valued, and you're going to do the same for them.

7. You want to share your life with them:

If you try a new restaurant or watch a preview of a great movie, you know that your person is the one with whom you want to experience it.

He's making you feel loved and secure," "You're able to be yourself and feel accepted. They're making you want to be your best self, and they're bringing that out in you." It won't even take you a millisecond to make a decision; your gut knows.

8. You're always honest with each other:

Whether they tell you when you're the best version of yourself or admit that they're the best version of yourself. "You want to know that you can be vulnerable and share with your partner the deep, scary stuff and then feel closer.

Chapter 6

Is He Committed to You or Not?

What is the sound signal of commitment?

It is crucial to properly "read" the signs of engagement in a potential long-term partner. Of course, this is most important before "settling" with someone, particularly if your partner wants to know the future of a relationship. You can press for this information too early, but you can also wait too long to clarify the big question: Is this person like me?

Well, I mean, the signal is valid. The message reflects something about engagement and is not just noise. Three critical features of ethical commitment signals are:

1. The behaviour is related to something about commitment:

Response matters a lot that you can judge a person with you from their behaviour; it doesn't mean you're starting to think about every single thing like saying, "I want to make a baby with you," without any other evidence of commitment like, say, marriage. If someone says to you, "I'd consider you to have my baby," an even worse indicator of commitment is. Context matters a lot here. It may sound stupid, but in some teenage groups, this is, in fact, a relatively common behaviour in which males tell females they are interested in some version of this. Some may be flattered and impressed, but in these examples, if someone said, "I want to raise a child with you," it would be much more impressive. That statement contains more information, especially if it is accurate, but that is the essence of engagement, which is about wanting and planning a future.

If a couple tells you they're married; you know a lot about their commitment. That doesn't mean that everything is excellent, of course. Similarly, if a couple tells you they're planning to get married, you can assume that there's a lot of commitment. I think even apart from marriage; a couple that says they have a lifetime commitment together tells you something important about a wedding.

2. The behaviour is controlled by the one who does it whatever it is:

For reaction to mean something about commitment, the individual has control over performing must be actioned. A shotgun wedding, for example, has less information about the participants ' level of commitment than other marriages, because the context limits one's options.

Similarly, if it is in the context of a hormonal rush of chemicals when the chemistry is driving the bus, "I love you" contains less information about commitment. Chemistry is fun, but it's not a great bus driver, and the windy mountain roads without guardrails are some relationships.

Mostly, when a person has options, the signals contain more information. If you have more choices, what you choose will tell you more about who you are. When a person has diminished options, less information about their exact preferences is contained in what they want.

Think about purchasing 7-Eleven toilet paper. It'll probably be a one-roll quantity brand, and it'll probably cost you four bucks. 7-Eleven is a great store chain, but they are excellent at convenience, not at low prices or varieties. What does it mean? If you need a roll of toilet paper badly, you should take the individually wrapped package of Scott's that they have and forego the ability to get the Charmin Ultra Soft that you usually prefer. (Which is my favourite at risk of oversharing.) How does this apply to date and matching? Anything that restricts your options, or that of your partner, restricts the information contained in your choices. That means some people can misinterpret their partners ' behaviour on a routine basis and think something can signal commitment if it doesn't. This also means that some couples who have been together for a while, with an unclear future, and who also have the constraints of living together may find it difficult to read in each other what they really want for the future.

3. A Small sacrifice can be the right signals of commitment:

Mean by sacrifice some extraordinary self-sacrifice feat. That would matter, of course, but it means little, daily indicators that a person is willing to put his partner or relationship first. And mean mutual sacrifice: There are two donors in a healthy relationship, each giving to each other and the involvement in small, meaningful ways.

If you see someone and think together about a future, ask yourself if you see evidence that they can sometimes put aside what they want for what's best for you.

In intimate relationships, there are several studies on sacrifice; I do not attempt here to cover that literature. But scholars have found and argued that certain types of sacrificial behaviour are reliable engagement indicators, such as

• Your man will sometimes change his schedule for you.

• Your man is going to do fun things he or she doesn't like as much as you do.

• Your man will appear early to help you prepare for a big event.

• Your companion will interrupt what he is doing to handle something that will bother you.

You're getting the idea. Of course, doing such things for your partner is just as important, but here I'm focused on you being able to read the level of commitment this person has to you.

The best signal is sometimes the one that shows that something is missing.

If you're looking for lasting love, challenge yourself to look for signs of love and commitment, that means something.

Yet note that sometimes love can be blind:

Some of you might be wise to ask trusted friends or family about what they see and what is important to them.

He Is Committed to You, Even If He Hasn't Said It Yet:

When you think you've found the person you'd like to commit to forever, you're probably pleased and excited.

That phase in a relationship where you have not yet fully discussed where you are, but you may know that the two of you are secure and in love is one of the most fun times in the life of a couple. While there may still be some confusion, which can make it even more exciting, there should also be a lot of happiness (hopefully) there.

But the answer may not always be that clear at times. You may be someone who respects verbal acknowledgment of commitment over anything else, or maybe the person you see may not be open about their emotions. Or, perhaps you're in a relationship happy and want a little more proof that your partner is ready to engage with you. Regardless, it's not uncommon to want to be sure that the person you love is committed to you.

All relationships are different, of course, and some people will vary in the way they show affection and commitment. I talk to an expert about the signs your partner is committed to, even though they may not say it, to get a general sense of some things to look out for.

1. You Are his Priority:

If he makes his girl the priority in his life, it's obvious when a man is dedicated. If they're putting you first, that's one of the most reliable signs they're dangerous. If he chooses to see you instead of spending time with his friends, you know things are going well, "if your partner spends all their time with other people and doesn't make time for you, they might not be ready for engagement.

It's even more certain that if they don't mind moving things around just getting to see you, they're committed.

2. You have the keys to the house:

"Once a man gives you the keys to the place where he lives, he is 100% committed to you. You'll admit that you avoided giving your keys to people at any cost in previous relationships. It was a private person who hated the idea that someone might drop by unannounced or unwanted. However, before you committed, your partner had keys to your house.

3. Remember the Little Things:

It's not about always the big things, like time together and space in the lives of each other.

Sometimes it's all about the little things, literally: "A loyal guy is one who listens to all you say, even if you don't think he's." It shows that it doesn't just mean that your partner listens to your big life plans. Instead, they'll know all about you literally, and they'll show you they're doing the things they're doing for you.

"He knows your favourite foods, places, and things, then goes out this way to make sure you get them. He'll do this because he wants you to feel happy and secure," "It might not be great gestures, but he'll surprise you by dropping back and forth in little reminders."

4. You are referred to as "we":

If your partner has already nestled comfortably in this active couple's life, they will call you a" we, "even if you don't know.

That occurs more obviously when they speak to those who matter about them: "Pay attention when you hear him talking with his friends and family. Is he referring to you as a partner? Maybe he will say something like' We'd love to come' without even mentioning an invite that might be for him." It's the times where they say something off-handily about the two of you being a team that you're thinking about. And be mindful that the opposite is also exact: if you believe you are a "we," and they're just considered alone, you might be heading for heartbreak.

5. He doesn't play Games:

To keep you hanging on, an immature person who isn't ready for a commitment will use stupid dating tricks and tactics. A mature, loving partner who is willing to be with you forever won't do anything like that.

"A genuine, committed man knows what he wants and is not afraid to go for it," "He doesn't try to test you and see if he can push your buttons or make you jealous. Then, he politely treats you and does everything he can to make you happy." It's not just because they want brownie points; it's because seeing you happy will make them happy too. A person who really wants to be committed to you will not risk playing games and losing you because, as "He knows what he has and does not intend to lose it!"

6. He Talks About the Future with You:

At all costs, a person who is not super engaged will avoid talking about the future. Before you committed, you may be someone who hated commitment, but when he's connected with you, it all changed, and he wanted to talk a lot about your future together.

If a person spontaneously speaks about your future together, it's a good sign that they're committed to you: "If he's serious about you, he won't be afraid to talk about where things might go." What he's talking about depends on where you're in your relationship, "If it's early, he might want to schedule a trip together, or if you've been together for a while, he might want to make sure you're on it, of course. If they do, and this is how you feel about them.

He's Only Committed to You

Every time when you enter a new relationship, you hope it's going to last. But a guy turns out to be a total dud every once in a while, and it blinds you. You are spending so much time trying to figure out if a guy is worth it or not, and it hurts when you really feel like he's, and then he turns around and screws up. That is not to be denied.

So, how do you see the true colours of a man in the world? Are there any signs of a sure-fire that he will not break your heart? Well, we can't predict the future, and with absolute certainty, you can never know whether a man is worth it or not. Relationships are always going to be difficult. People can change and do all the time, and you can do nothing to fix it. But there are definitely a few tell-tale signs that you and only you are committed to a guy! It doesn't mean your relationship is going to be perfect or last forever, but it does mean you can trust that it won't throw you out of the blue or cheat on you. Here are clear signs that he is only committed to you.

1. Take On a Real Date:

Going on real "dates" these days are becoming rarer and rarer. So many relationships start as a situation of "friends with benefits," and on a real date, the guy will never end up asking the girl. Now, you should go for it if you want to go ahead and ask a guy first on a date! Nothing will deter you. But if you want to see whether or not a guy is really in you, give him a little time to ask you on a date. It doesn't have to be a fancy dinner and a film, but something that shows real planning beyond, "Hey, my friend is having a party, come through." A guy is more committed to making an effort to decide on a plan and treat you to a nice date.

2. Trust You with His Phone:

So many couples are fighting on social media these days. It can start a lot of drama. Technology also makes it easier to be sly and talk behind your back to an ex or another person. It's enough to make a girl feel like she's going to have to sleep with one eye open and make sure her man doesn't act shady all the time! But there are some good guys out there who are still going to be faithful. If a guy is completely cool to borrow his mobile and doesn't bother to hide anything on it, it's always a good sign. This means he doesn't have anything to hide. And if a guy knows his phone password very well, it's even better. An honest man will not bother to hide his messages.

3. Introduce You to His Family

Many guys are not trying to introduce girls to their families these days. That's because dating is so casual that people don't think it's a big deal. But frankly, in any relationship, it is a very important step. It means the guy cares about you enough to introduce you in his life to the other important people. It also means he wants you to like his family! When a man introduces you to his family, it means that in his life, he considers you to be a very special person. If he saw you as a casual hook up, believe us, he wouldn't bring you to his parents for dinner! This is a definite sign of commitment.

4. Traveling together with you:

Planning a trip together is a big step for any couple. While traveling, it's so easy for things to go wrong. You might end up getting into dumb fights over small mistakes, you have to stick together and sort out things like finding your way in an unfamiliar place, and at some point, and you will probably end up feeling hungry, cranky, and jet-lagged. But if a man wants to travel with you and you manage to get along during the trip, find him engaged! It means he's willing to plan with you to make sure you both have a good time, save a decent amount of money to spend on a trip with you, and want to experience the best of life with you by his side.

5. Encourage You to Have a Girls ' Night:

Some guys get very jealous when you want to spend time away from him with your own mates. Isn't this the worst thing? It's not good to be attached to the hip all the time for a couple. Everybody needs their own room, as well as their own group of friends. If a man is possessive of you and you don't want to spend time with your girlfriends, he may have some insecurity issues and may not be the best guy to date. But if you're actually encouraged by a guy to spend quality time with your friends and have some independence, this is a really good sign. This indicates he's spending time apart completely comfortable and believes you're honest with him.

6. Memorize Your Coffee Order:

Small stuff, right? It's always a pleasant surprise when a guy knows what you need, right when you need it. Moreover, anyone who takes the time to memorize small details about you is usually a guardian. It shows they pay attention to the small things that may not be noticed by other people. Every girl now has a usual order of coffee. Whether you like cappuccinos or macchiato or you're always looking for lattes of pumpkin spice (even in the summer), you probably know your "normal" heart. If a man learns your usual order of coffee and surprises you with it every once in a while, it means that he is careful enough to notice the little things you enjoy. It's a sure sign he's falling in love with!

7. Go Shopping with You:

Well, what kind of guy would you consider to go shopping? Is it a myth? Okay, let's make it clear that a good boyfriend might not want to go shopping with you, but sometimes he'll do it anyway. Guys may not enjoy shopping as much as girls do, and it's not like you'd like to drag him along on every shopping trip, but if a guy goes shopping with you every once in a while without complaining seriously, consider it a win. We all know guys don't really like going shopping, but the point here is that he's doing something fun with you just because you are enjoying it, even though it's not his favourite thing in the world. It's a sweet gesture, and if it wasn't committed, he wouldn't.

8. Make plans for the future

Here's a big one! A guy who is not committed to you is not going to make any serious plans for the future. He may, for instance, reflect ongoing one day to a certain restaurant or on a road trip, but he will never make any concrete plans. But a guy who really loves you will think far ahead because he expects to be with you from now on for months and months. He won't hesitate to say you're supposed to plan anything six months from today or even suggest going to an event that's not going to happen for another year because, at that stage, he just wants to be with you. A man who refuses to make real plans for the future is not a man with whom to live!

9. Write You Love Letters:

This event is so sweet, old-fashioned. In the days of Tinder and other dating apps, it is definitely not very common, but there are still guys who are going to do it! If a man ever writes a letter of love to you, it means he's for you head over heels! This is something so sweet and romantic for a woman to do. It's a guarantee he's great in you. No man who sees you as a casual fling would ever have taken the time and effort to write a letter of love. It's just not true. The same man who is writing to you at 3 a.m. doesn't sit down to write a letter of love. Nope, the kind of guy who sends a letter of love is the kind of guy that really cares.

10. Invite You to Hang Out with His Friends:

Recall when earlier we said that if a man is okay with you making plans with your girlfriends and not including him, does that mean that he feels secure and committed in your relationship? Okay, if he invites you to hang out with him and his family, which means he wants you to be part of his inner circle. Many guys get annoyed if their girlfriends try to join while they're hanging out with their friends, but if sometimes a guy is happy to get you tagged along, it's a positive sign. Keeping a balance in your relationships is crucial. For instance, you want to be able to hang out with friends of each other and your own groups— you need some friends of each other and some independence.

11. Note when you get a haircut:

Men are usually completely blind to a girl who gets a new haircut. How many times did you get a haircut or even have your hair coloured, happy to show it to your guy and get a compliment, just to keep him completely silent when you walked in the room? Yeah, it's common knowledge that when we get out of haircut, men don't seem to notice. But if you find a guy who really takes note of those tiny details, when you get your haircut, he'll definitely give you a compliment! He may not notice a little trim, of course, but he will say something if you look good. So take note of those guys who say something after you've got a haircut.

12. Hold Your Hand in Public:

Some men don't like the public showing off their girlfriends. Yeah, what's that? You should be absolutely proud to be with her if you're dating. You should be able to walk hand in hand down the street, so everyone can look at you and think, "Wow, who is the lucky man? "If a man refuses to hold his hand in public, that's why. There's something going on. Maybe he doesn't want that other woman to know about he's in a relationship because he still wants their attention, or maybe he's confused with being with you, but he doesn't want to be alone. It's so confusing! He would be happy to hold your hand all the time if he is truly committed to you.

13. Send You Little Reminders:

There's nothing sweeter than the same guy's constant "good morning" and "good evening" send! It means that when he wakes up and the last thing at night before he falls asleep, he thinks of you first thing in the morning. But it's even nicer to have a guy who goes beyond that and sends you sweet little reminders. For example, sending you a text to drive safely because he knows you've got a long drive ahead, wishing your parents or siblings a happy birthday, letting you know he saw something that reminded him of you — all these would be good signs. Again, remembering those little things is all about. That's what a partnership at the end of the day really keeps going.

14. Say "I Love You" First:

When a guy first says, "I love you," it's definitely a big deal! That's the funny thing about relationships men are normally expected to ask the girl first, but as we see girls as being more emotional than guys, most guys are going to hesitate to say "I love you" before their girlfriend does. So if a guy decides to let down his guard and take that first step by saying those three small words, it's a great sign for you. This means he's all right when you see him weak. This means he trusts you, as he knows that you won't exploit him or violate his feelings for you after you hear those words. This is one of the clearest signs that he is actually committed to.

15. Give You Homemade Gifts:

Homemade gifts mean a lot more than store gifts bought! Now, this doesn't mean you're not loved by a guy if he buys you gifts from the stores you like. But it is worth holding on to a guy who puts extra effort into creating something for you. This shows he's willing to put time and energy into creating something special and unique for you alone. Many people don't come into contact with their creative side, which is a real shame. But it's definitely a special guy who goes out of his way to make something handmade for you! The gifts he gives you are going to be keepsakes you can hold on to represent together your great memories forever.

The Biggest Sign He Will Never Be Committed to you:

He never shares secrets of anything profound about himself with you:

A commitment to sharing things is the most important; if a person does not tell you about their secrets or doesn't want to share ideas with you, then he does not wish to any commitment with you.

He won't introduce you to his family:

The person who loves you and wants that you become the part of his life will like to present you with his family and friends; if your man feel hesitation while doing this it's mean that he is not committed to you truly

He tells you he's not looking for a relationship the person who doesn't need contact with you, try to make arguments with you on small things and every time he tells you that he does not want to live with you because he doesn't want to make any commitment with you

He doesn't make any effort to reach you:

A person who loves you, want to meet you at your free time, try to make efforts and go out with you because he wants to spend time with you, but the person who is not committed to you does not make any efforts for you because he doesn't want any commitment with you.

He only calls you late at night:

In mostly relationship the guy who loves you try to talk with you or want to spend their free time with you, on the other side the men who do not want any commitment try to ignore you and only try to talk with you when they are free most probably at night

He never gets jealous:

A man who truly loves you get suspicious from another guy when they try to get closer to you, and its human nature, but the men who are not committed to you does not bother this and try to avoid the things

He's not giving you time in his life:

Relationships need time if two people spend a lot of time together, one of the very first signs of engagement in a relationship. Outside of regular working hours, there is generally not much time left to spare with all the things you could do in a day. And since time is one of the few resources that none of us can get back, it is a good sign that you and your significant other choose to make time for each other regularly. If your man is not giving you time, it means that he is not committed to you.

In the big decisions he makes, he doesn't include you:

"If your partner makes important life decisions without thinking about you and it affects your relationship, that should tell you that your relationship is not a priority for the big decisions like that are something that should be addressed together, mainly when one partner is away for a specified period. It's essential to be a supportive partner, but it's just as necessary to keep up with it. If your man isn't discussed with you while making important decisions, you don't matter to him, and he doesn't want to engage with you.

He's not over his ex:

When a guy is not emotionally over his ex, this will become an issue for you.

The problem with most men is that they will deny, deny, deny that they still have feelings for their ex even when you ask them directly. And it defiantly affects your relationship; if your man still loves his ex, he is not able to make a new relationship or commitment with you.

Here are few Signs Those Mean He is Not Serious About You

1. He Flakes On You All The Time:

It means you are important to him when a guy is serious about you. For what he said he was going to do, he's going to follow through. What's the reason? Well, when a guy takes a woman seriously, he hopes she will feel the same way about him. He knows she would give up on him and move on if he treats her like she is unimportant or flakes on her a lot. So he's making it his priority to keep going with her. Whether he flakes on you all the time or cancels at the last minute, that means he's not too concerned about your feelings, which is a big sign that he's not so serious about you.

2. He's not letting himself be open to you:

Being open to someone else takes trust. This means that if you are at your most insecure, you trust them not to reject you. All partners are confident to be open to each other in any good relationship—since they respect each other. But it can be frightening to be safe with someone different. If he's never open around you—if he's always wearing a "mask" or never really allowing himself to be vulnerable, that means he is too nervous for being with you, or he doesn't think it's worth it. If you're at the very beginning of your relationship, it's not a big deal, but if you've been together long enough to open up now and he doesn't, it's a sign he's not all that serious.

3. He doesn't want you to meet his friends or family:

When there's a close relationship between two people, they don't just date each other. We share their lives, as well. And that means sharing the people near you. Meeting the friends of your significant other, and finally, parents is a classic step in any relationship. These are the people he thinks most of, and they are the ones he most values for their views. He's going to want you to meet his friends and family if he's serious about you, not only to show them who he's dating but also so you can see that side of him and get closer as a couple. When he keeps you away from his friends and family, it's a sign that he doesn't want you

4. Around each other, you don't feel comfortable:

Good relationships are all about intimacy. And intimacy can only develop when two people have sufficient trust in each other to be truly vulnerable. If it doesn't feel comfortable to be with him, or when he's with you, he doesn't seem happy, it's a huge barrier to a deeper friendship and intimacy between you. Good, lasting relationships exist when you can be around someone else, and they can be around you, without any fear of rejection. If being together isn't easy; it's a sign you may not be compatible with each other, which is a major sign that things won't get serious.

5. He Doesn't Make Time for You:

I spoke a little earlier about this, but it bears repeating: if a man is serious about you, then you become important to him. You are becoming one of his goals. That's not to suggest he'll drop it all and spend 100% of his time with you. It simply means that he will treat you as needed and make an effort to spend time with you and balance his life with a commitment to you in it. So if he's still busy, or he never really has time to be with you, it's a big sign that he doesn't treat you as an important part of his life because he doesn't take you seriously.

6. He's not curious about who you are:

If he thinks things could get complicated and he's worried about you, he'll want to know all he can find out about who you are.

Why? Because he wants to know what that future will hold if he sees a potential future with you!

He'll be interested in what makes you tick, who you're under the mask, who you're like a person, so he'll be able to figure out how far he'll see things going between you.

When, while you're dating, he doesn't even have the desire to find out anything about you, it means that isn't that important to him, which is another massive sign that he isn't serious about you.

7. You Never Make Future Plans Together:

These need not necessarily be huge plans like the relationship's future or something like that. It can be as simple as inviting a birthday party a month in advance, or something like that, for this example. A guy who doesn't want to plan with you in the future and just hangs out every day is a guy who isn't so serious about the relationship. So if all of your dates and hangouts start from a text and happen that night, if you're never planning to do anything a week or a month ahead of time, it's really not that serious about you.

8. Your Gut Is Telling You He's not:

The best guide in your love life will be your intuition. If your heart is screaming at you trying to make you believe something, your gut will be a much better guide as to whether it is true. You're here because you're looking for signs to confirm what's true you're hoping for. Perhaps you're hoping he's serious about you, and you're looking for signs to confirm that assumption. Take the time to ask yourself if you really think he's serious, and honestly answer yourself. The sudden feeling in your stomach will give you a better response than hours of rationalization about it.

9. He doesn't want his girlfriend to call you:

This one is quite obvious. If he doesn't want to call you his wife or mark the relationship, it's a pretty big indication that he isn't that serious. Guys want to avoid names when they're not in a relationship and want the status quo to be maintained. An uninterested guy will try to shut it down as quickly as possible as soon as they feel a demand for a relationship tag. What's the reason? Since he likes things just as they are and because he's not all that serious about the relationship in the first place, he doesn't want them to advance any further.

10. He Doesn't Trust You:

Trust is the most important aspect of any partnership. You need to trust each other in order to be vulnerable and open, to have confidence in each other, and to have the strength to nurture and support each other. Without confidence, none of a good relationship's intimacy and closeness will develop. And you know, if you trust him in your heart, and if he trusts you, you will feel. It's easy to tell if there's confidence in a relationship when you're honest with yourself or you're not. Trust takes time to grow, so don't be afraid if you've just started dating and still don't trust each other deeply. But if you have been dating for a while, and they still are, there is no real trust between you. Unfortunately, it's a big sign that the relationship isn't serious.

11. He says He doesn't want any serious thing:

It seems this should be a visible sign, but it's not. Most guys are going to tell a woman they don't want anything serious, but then they're going to give her an excuse.

"I don't want anything serious right now."· "I don't want anything serious while I'm looking for a job."· "I don't want anything serious because I'm not over my ex yet." The issue is that when a guy does that, most people hear the part of the reason yet totally ignore the part of "I don't want something serious" when that's what the guy said.

Your man is only your man!

The man who loves you is only yours, no one takes your place in his life, and through his actions, and you can understand this. Here are the few signs that he loves you and never wants you to suffer, don't stress about the situation, he still shows you love and care by his actions.

He's holding your hand:

A man who only wants his body won't hold your hand. It's a sign he wants to say you're his beloved to the world. If he does it when you're on your own, it's apparent that he always needs to be next to you.

Talking of cute expressions:

There is nothing more personal and sweet than the kisses of the forehead. There is no desire for it;

there is no ulterior motive. Just a simple gesture, affectionate and somewhat protective.

He often laughs when he's with you:

When you're just too relaxed within, do you feel like you're going to burst? And you're just grinning like a fool; you can't stop? When he's around you, that's how he thinks.

He can't keep his hands off you:

Does he always manage to reach you in a small way? A hand on your waist or back, an arm around your shoulder, a defensive arm on your knee?

He introduces you to mom:

When a man willingly, uncorked, and unprovoked decides to take you home to meet mom, you earned. You have my compliments! Unless they're serious about the gal, men don't waste time with this.

He introduces you to the "gang":

The person who is committed to you and wants you in his life give you priority; he adds you with his friends and family because he needs you for lifetime

In his kisses:

Kissing is not reserved for people in love, but there is a gap between a lustful kiss and a caring one. If he can't get enough of your lips and gets kissing you, even without sex, there's a pretty good chance you got him hooked.

He is listening to you:

You know the irritating things men are doing where you're talking, and they ignore you and sometimes throw in an absent-minded "Uh-huh?" He's not doing that for you. He appears to be interested in what you're saying by god and doesn't tune you out.

He speaks about the future:

When a man fears commitment or does not plan to stick around, he does not map with you. So, if he's alluded together to your future, it's a sign that he thinks you're a guardian.

He calls "just because":

A sign that he often thinks of you is that without a specific reason, he calls or texts. He wants to see how you are, listen to your voice, and speak a little to you. If you didn't occupy his mind, he wouldn't feel the need.

You're making him laugh:

The more he thinks about you, the more he likes you. He thinks you're the best, and what shouldn't you love?

He's making time for you:

We're all swamped, and time is precious. However, he chooses to spend the time with you, and often. That's saying something. You're a priority for him.

He misses you:

The behaviour of a man, when you're not around, is just as important as that in your presence. Is he thinking of you? Are you always telling him to miss you? If you're not there, is there a hole in his life? It means that you have become a part of him successfully.

He is standing up taller:

If he's standing up a little straight, a little taller when you're around, he wants to impress you and make you look attractive. It's sweet.

He gives you gifts that mean something:

On our first birthday, my boyfriend gave me a first edition of "Love in Cholera Time;" he remembered that I quoted it on our first date. You see, anyone can buy expensive jewellery, but to give you something valuable, it takes a particular person.

That's right. He's domestic:

If he switches from bars and drinks to staying at home and cooking with you, that's something to be taken into consideration. If he'd rather be old and lazy with you on the sofa than go out with his mates, that's a love statement right there.

With your kids:

Not only is he not bothered that you have a past and a family, but he actively embraces his role in their lives. He always brings something to your kids and enjoys spending time with them. Isn't this just making you swoon?

He's a bit nervous about you:

When men are shy, especially when they blush, it's always nice. He likes you because you make him excited.

He turns to look at you frequently:

Does he turn around to look at you, even if he does anything different? Does he look up to smile at you from his phone? Check what you're doing? When talking to friends, catch your eye across the bar? You know the meaning of that.

He praises your personality:

Saying you're warm is nice, but what makes your heart melt is when he reveals how much he loves your sense of humour or childish laughter.

With you, he inconveniences himself:

Helping you out is not always easy, and sometimes it also requires something that he hates. But he does it anyway because it's for you and because he loves you, please, because of* drumroll*.

He's still doing beautiful things for you:

Someone interested in and involved with their spouse can find ways for them to do beautiful things. Breakfast in bed, when he comes home from work, buying chocolate, or even just a backrub when you're in your time.

He stands up for you:

It goes without saying that if you are not treated correctly, a man who loves you will protect you fiercely and stand up for you. Be proud of that!

He's staying the night:

If he's interested in just sex, he's going to make any excuse to get the hell out after the deed is over. But if he's staying, he's more than just being sexually released.

He supports you:

A kind and loving spouse, whatever they may be, support your dreams and actions, and even if it means that he will see you less or if he disagrees. It is not just a sign of maturity; it is a sign of love.

He gives you space:

Love doesn't mean to kill your friend! Love is sometimes found between two partners in the vacuum. He understands that you need it and, unprompted, he gives it to you.

He's putting you first:

A famous verse says love is selfless, and that's true. If even to his detriment, he puts you first, then there is no real question about it.

He's comfortable at your place:

Trekking to your home and spending time there, he likes it. Hell, even an extra set of PJs and a toothbrush has been brought. For the long haul, the man is here.

He's sharing stuff with you:

He doesn't like to open up about personal things, but it's different with you. He knows you're never going to judge him, and he can be vulnerable around you, which is one of the biggest compliments he can give you.

He picks up on your behaviours:

Did you know that loving couples tend to mirror the behaviour of each other? And it's amazing.

He lets you win:

Listen, people like winning. They are what they are doing; they are winners. So, admitting someone else is right, or even literally allowing someone else to succeed in a game, cost them their ego. And, because he loves you, he will gladly give it to you.

He's just a bit jealous:

You're him, and he won't share you with anyone. Not in a possessive manner, only in a loving way that says he's here for a long time, exclusively, and he wants you to be too.

Chapter 7

Best Words About Love, Commitment and Relationship

Love's best and worst thing is that it can't be conveyed in words:

It may be challenging to express those feelings into words when you love someone. Yes, true love can make you feel weak in your knees and unable to speak. Maybe that's the best kind of love where the other person makes you fall in love so thoroughly that you can't think appropriately, although it can also become a problem.

This list of all time's best love quotes will surely make it easier for your partner to express your emotions and feelings of love. Such famous quotes and expressions of inspiring love will allow you to explain precisely how you feel with the most straightforward wording.

Throughout this, you will find quotes from this generation as well as from previous productions.

But each of these quotes is created by someone who, at one point or another, was deeply in love.

So, here are the best phrases about love and being in love, you can use to express your feelings to your partner without any further do.

Inspirational Love Quotes and Sayings

• When I'm next to you, I'm happy:

If you're in love with true love, you'll know that this person will complete you and make you happy when you're together. Never let them go once you find this person!

"Water only shines through the sun. And you are my sun."

• Because of you, my night has become sunny dawn:

If your partner lights up your heart, no matter how dark your day is, then this is the perfect quote of love for them.

"I swear I couldn't love you more than I do now, yet I know I'm going to love you tomorrow."

• You may hold my hand for a while, but you're holding my heart forever:

This quote of love indicates that love has no constraints or time limits. It's sporadic and real. Even if you may not spend eternity in the arms of your mate, you may still keep them forever in your heart.

"There's a folly in loving you, a lack of reason that makes you feel so flawless."

• I know I am in love with you because, finally, my reality is better than my dreams:

A well-known quote on love tells us that true love, including your dreams, will feel better than anything else. When in your daily life you can be happier than in your dreams, you've found the one.

"Before I want to sleep, you are the last thought in my mind and the first thought when I wake up every morning."

• I need you as a heart needs a rhythm:

This quote will melt your partner's soul. We all know, of course, that your heart needs a beat to live, and if you share these quotes of love with your partner, you tell them that without them, your life is meaningless. That quote about love is so deep and meaningful, and it will help you to convey the feelings of true love.

"You know it's love when you want that person to be happy, even if you're not part of their happiness."

• All I need to feel is your affection:

Did you feel totally in love with your partner? Would your life feel incomplete without them?

Then this couple love quotes is the one you need to share with your partner to help explain exactly how you feel.

• Until the stars go out, I'll love you, and the tides don't turn:

That quote is relatively self-explanatory, and you're not going to stop loving your partner. No matter what's going on. It doesn't matter how things end. Your love will last for eternity. For her, these romantic quotes will surely set off those emotions of love.

• Stay and pay no rent in my heart:

You don't care about things that are mundane or how much your partner has to offer. Everything you know is that you love them and pledge to give them your soul.

• I fall in love again every time I see you:

Every day you fall deeper in love, no matter how new or old your relationship is. If you have a partner who makes you feel this way, be sure to share with them this beautiful quote of love and never let them out of

• You're my album. You're my love song:

Always feel like your partner must remind you of every love song, or will you make a love song just for them? That brief quote of love would then be the perfect expression of your affection.

• It's because of you if I know what love is:

This quote of love helps us to understand what we feel when we fall in love. The only reason you know what love is or what it feels is because of your partner, and you should let them know by sharing with them the best quote of love.

• Our friendship is meant to be something in the stars that have been written and drawn into our destiny:

This romantic quote on love will help you set the mood by letting them know exactly how you feel about your relationship when you think you've finally found your soul mate. It may have taken some time to meet and fall in love with both of you. But once you've done that, it's clear that you were both meant to be together.

• I realized that the first time you met me, I was destined to be yours:

If you have that bond with your partner that you know you can't ignore, this is the kind of inspiring quote of love that you should give them. It's just like saying you were meant to be together, and from the beginning, you knew it.

"It's part of living a balanced life to lose balance for love at times."

• Let's Flip the coin and see. Head, I belong to you. You are mine, tail. Yeah, we're not going to lose:

You and your partner will always share a deep love connection with each other, regardless of what happens in life or what obstacles are thrown your way. Share this lovely quote with your partner to let them know you're always going to love them no matter what.

• There's Happiness where there's Love:

The love of your life is your partner, and there's no better way to put it. They give you a reason for living and a reason for the happy living once you've found a person who gives you that feeling, be sure to let them know how loved they are and how lucky you're both to observe this kind of love.

"Love is a disease. At any happen to anyone at any time. "

There is only happiness in life, love, and love:

This quote of love defines love as true happiness in the purest form. With overwhelming respect for you, this single sentence will have your partner weak in the knees.

• I can't do anything without his love; there's nothing I can do with his love:

Once you meet the one person that completes your life, their love can make you feel you can do anything. It'll make you feel powerful and unlimited. It is a once-in-a-lifetime experience to find such a love. This is one of the best quotes that I love you; you'll ever see.

"Love is like the wind, you can't see it, but you can hear it,"

• No one can make me weightless and carefree as you can:

If the love of your partner makes you feel lovely and carefree, you've met your match. Make sure to let them know how you think by sharing this. I love you to quote with them and how they make you feel.

• It was never a choice to love you. It's been a must:

If love is real and destined to be accurate, then you're not going to have an option to fall. You will have the weakest form of love in the knees and come to you when you least expect it. If love feels compelled, it might not be accurate.

• Just when I think you can't love you anymore, you're proving me wrong:

You may know you love your partner as much as you can, but every new morning gives you a more profound sense of love for them. This quote on love will explain your deepest desire.

• It's true that when you take my name, my heart still skips a beat:

This saying of love perfectly explains how true love feels. Next to what this unique form of love feels, passion and desire is nothing? This quote of perfect love will help you to explain your love to your partner correctly.

• All my life, I loved you; it took me so long to find you:

This is the best being in quotes of love to have love and affection for your partner. Finding your perfect partner may have taken you a while, but you knew all along that you loved them dearly and have an immediate connection.

• Love is when the happiness of the other person is more significant than yours:

One of the best love sayings. Marriage is everything about sacrifices and compromises. It means putting your partner's feelings before your own, without purpose at times. But it becomes the most accurate form of love when you both do this in your relationship.

• You don't know how difficult it is to force myself sometimes to stop thinking about you:

It sometimes becomes impossible to stop thinking about our partner when we fall in love. Let them know how much you feel throughout the day about their devotion by dedicating to them this loving quote.

• It is not possible to blame gravity for falling in love:

That quote shows how uncontrollable it is to fall in love. This is one of the best love saying that lovers around the world will share for decades to come.

"Falling in love is simple. The hardest part is finding someone to hold you."

• I want to live a hundred minus one day if you live to be a hundred, so I never have to live without you:

That beautiful quote of love shows how much you love your partner. So much, that without them you wouldn't want to spend a day of your life. Isn't it just a sweet and lovely word about love?

• Sex soothes tension. It's the cause of love:

This quote is quite self-explanatory. Loving produces the best of memories and feelings. This is one of the quotes from great love.

• If you look at him, the best attitude is, and he's already looking:

How wonderful is it to look at your partner and discover that you are already being admired? If this makes you feel like your friend, be sure to let them know.

• You may be one person to the universe, but you're the world for one person:

Your partner's love should make you feel like you're the world's only one. When they make you feel good, make sure you tell them to pledge this love.

·It is dying of blindness, errors, and treason:

True love is never going to die. But if love is not real, it will end only when there are betrayal and unbearable pain. Ideally, with your current lover, you will never have to feel this pain.

• Love is better than an obligation as an educator.

Love is going to teach you things nothing else can do. It's going to show you comfort and pain. But above all, it's going to teach you how to live.

• I knew you were excellent, and I loved you. Then I saw you were not perfect, and even more, I loved you:

No one is perfect. And you shouldn't ask for an ideal lover. Yet embrace your partner and learn to love their faults as they are.

Here, we found the best quotes for your commitment to keep your eyes open (and melt your heart in the process).

1. "I started to search for you the minute I heard my first love story, not knowing how blind I was. Ultimately, lovers don't meet anywhere. Everywhere they are in one another. "

2. " True love is selfless. It is ready to sacrifice. "

3. " A successful marriage requires many times, falling in love, always with the same person."

4. " Having a caring and committed heart toward someone a heart so steadfast in its devotion that, despite the state of health, appearance, reputation, finances, troubles, or challenges that, dear world, is love, the object of its desire should be neglected."

5. "What a nice and holy fashion is that those who love one another can rest on the same bed."

6. "I mean, if the marriage cannot survive the long term, why would it be worth my time and energy for the short term on Earth?"

7. "Today, I missed you. You still love it. It's always there."

8. "The satisfaction of a relationship can be measured by the number of bruises each partner bears on their tongues, received from years of biting back angry words."

9. "Nothing is worse than being apart," I don't care how hard it is to be together."

10. "Love is an unconditional devotion to an imperfect person. It's not just a strong feeling to love someone. It's a choice, a determination, and a promise."

11. "Finally, it became clear to her that love was not about finding someone to marry perfectly. Love was about seeing a person's truth and accepting all their shades of light and darkness."

12. "If you're not too long, I'm going to wait for you all my life."

13. "Love is not the greatest emotion."

14. "You need only one man to love you. But he's free to love you like a flame, mad like the stars, always like tomorrow, unexpectedly like an inhaler, and as the tides. Just one guy and all this."

15. " I can't explain to you how happy I am for our little infinity. "

16. " Relationships last forever because two people have chosen: KEEP IT. FIGHT FOR IT. AND WORK FOR IT. "

17. True stories of love never end.

Some of the famous sayings regarding an ideal man:

• The Ideal Man should speak to us like goddesses and treat us like children. He should refuse all our severe demands and gratify all our whims. He should encourage us to be capricious and prohibit us from having missions. He should always say a lot more than he means, and always mean a lot more than he says.

• There is no ideal man like that. The ideal man at the moment is the man that you love.

• The perfect man is happy to do things for others.

• Sting is my perfect man because he's a real man.

• The ideal man is a mate of his own and respects confidentiality.

• There's no ideal man. Having a husband is better.

• My perfect man is old white dead and on a green paper plate.

• I think that we have set our ideal on the wrong objects; I think that the greatest ideal man is self-perfection.

• Each time a guy stands up for an ideal or works to improve a lot of others or hits against injustice, a tiny ripple of hope is sent out.

• Up to that time, I had never known that I had any particular talent for discovery, but Lord Rayleigh, whom I always considered to be an ideal scientist, had said so, and if that were the case, I thought that I should focus on some great idea.

• My interpretation of the ideal man is' the particular man with whom, at that particular time, a woman is in love.

• Everything that the soul knows how to do can't fail to get.

• Good mental health, such as equality, is only available for one person if it exists for all.

• Many people carry in their minds an ideal man and woman, and when ordinary realistic interactions between men and women are debated in regard only to these unrealistic concepts, we should not be surprised by any ridiculous conclusions.

• "One of the qualities of the ideal man is in the superiority of self-control."

•To ask of men that they are bad is to say that they are worse than we think they are, or worse than the ideal man whose picture we have built on the basis of a few.

"Repentance is the perfect man's greatest punishment."

The ideal man carries with dignity and grace the mistakes of nature, making the best of circumstances.

My ideal man is loyal, trustworthy, and a gentleman who is capable of treating women.

"The only real reason certain relationships and marriages have not yet come to an end is that one of the spouses has not yet met their ideal partner or someone they love or at least like in every case."

Chapter 8

How Can You Keep Your Man?

How can you keep your man?

And you found the right thing, your dream man. You think he's the one with which you want to spend the rest of your life.

You think he's your soul mate or God's one for you. Having him by your side, you feel blessed. Having him is one of life's most significant accomplishments.

But it's great to have someone to hold him. The latter requires a great deal of confidence and commitment.

There are ways to keep him if you've found the right guy.

1. Trust him with your whole heart:

If you want to keep your kid, don't just treat him like another guy who doesn't trust him. Because of the gathered knowledge that men could not be trusted, most girls don't trust men. Not only will it make him feel unique and distinct from other guys if you believe your man, but it will make you unique in his eyes as well.

2. Be afraid to lose him:

If you want to keep your guy, don't behave like it's all right to lose him. Treasure him and make him feel valued. Show him how much in your life you want him to be held. But don't make it too much for you to become too insecure and possessive, of course.

3. Love yourself:

If you want to keep your man, show him that his presence in your life gives you growth and goodness. Don't hurt and blame him for the damage.

4. Have faith in it:

If you want to keep your guy, trust him. Believe it. Believe in it. Make him feel reliable and trustworthy. Either way, he's the man.

5. Make him feel good about it:

If you want to keep your man, don't make him feel bad about it. Let him know you are drawn to him sexually and to him alone. Surely some unique interest will make him stick with you.

6. Feel him the only one:

If you want to keep your guy, never cheat or even think of cheating. Men protect their egos so severely that they may also want to leave a woman ahead of time before they even cheat if they feel they're likely to do it.

7. Do not make him feel jealous either:

If you want to keep your guy, do not make him feel insecure. Don't do stupid things like orchestrating some act to make you happy and show your affection. Jealousy is a heart and brain pain. If they become jealous, do you think men like it? The reply is NO!

8. Let him know you:

If you want to keep your man, let him see through your heart and mind. Be honest and clear. Tell him when he politely asks you. It's not that he has no faith in you, but it's because he's always trying to build his confidence in you.

9. Be humble:

If you want to keep your man, get rid of your pride, learn to acknowledge your mistakes, and ask forgiveness. It's not cool and cute to get mad at him as a defensive strategy to cover up your sins. It's ridiculous and annoying.

10. Make sacrifices:

If you want to keep your guy, make him feel his true love. True love is known when you first think of him before yourself when you become selfless. It's going to make him realize you're a long-term woman to hold.

11. Be calm and patient:

Learn how to control your anger and manage your tantrums if you want to keep your man. You're not a nagger. Who can live with a nagger in a house?

12. Just be beautiful:

If you're going to keep your guy, be pleasing in your face, mind, and heart. By his interpretation, be fair. Consider the first time that made him fall in love with you. It could be your long hair, your sweet smile, or just your attitude.

13. Have an intimate relationship with him:

If you want to have your guy, don't let others dictate things in your relationship. Let the two of you determine your relationship's best, your marriage. Try to solve them on your own without allowing other people to interfere with it if there are problems or fighting within it.

14. Be affectionate with him:

If you want to keep your spouse, offer him the love he deserves. Guys need a warm feeling of not being cold and alone.

15. Be responsible:

If you want to keep your man, let him know you're ready for the future. Show yourself to be a mature woman, his children's responsible girlfriend, wife, or mother.

16. Protect it:

If you want to keep your man away from harm. Men also have vulnerabilities and need their wife's safety. As a woman, by offering him your guiding light, you can shield him from the darkness. Know how to console him if he's tired and sad. Men would probably remain with a woman who could have a relationship between two souls to love, protect, and support each other.

How to stay a man in love with you?

The kind of love that every day deepens among you. Wherever in the partnership, you are both happy, no matter what.

The kind of love you never again have to question the relationship where you believe he will love you until the end of time.

Here's the truth: to the ends of the earth, he may love you, but that doesn't guarantee that you will never again doubt the relationship. It just doesn't work to try to remove all questions from a relationship.

I know it sucks when things get tight between you, but there's no perfect relationship. Every relationship will have its ups and downs, even between two people who love each other to death.

If you put together two people who are right for each other, love will flourish. It's all about creating the best atmosphere between you to grow in love.

How would you make love grow among yourselves and make it that kind of love that remains high even in challenging times? And how do you keep the love going, also if you're a long-distance away from each other, so keep both people happy in the relationship, so it's going away?

1. Make sure you're at ease with each Other:

Mutual trust is the most critical factor in whether love is going to grow and whether a partnership is going to go away. The relationship won't last if you're not happy with each other. If you're not supposed to be hard with great relationships, they're meant to be easy. Being around him should feel good just like being around; you should feel good for him. When you're with each other, it feels good, and it's easy to be with each other, then you're happy. There are battles in all relationships. When you put two people together, it's inevitable, and they have to make compromises to move forward. How you fight is the difference between a great relationship and one that won't last. Should you break down and attack each other when you fight, or do you get to the bottom of what you're fighting for?

Right, happy partners don't try to hurt each other as they struggle; they try to solve everything they struggle and stop fighting. Couples that aren't compatible will mean they'll keep a fight going to get the last word in or "win back the other guy" for something they've said. Compatible couples will always glance to finish a fight, and that's what makes their relationships strong enough to distance themselves. No relationship can last without being compatible. The infatuation you feel for one another will eventually fade at the beginning of the relationship, and you'll wind up falling apart. So to make sure compatibility is the very first step in finding true love that lasts.

2. Be One That He Can Confide in:

To build a long-lasting, deep bond with you, he must feel like he can tell you anything. And stuff you may not want to learn.

The most important thing to create that bond is to make him feel secure when he tells you things. This means not punishing him for telling you the truth about something, and if he tells you something you don't want to hear, it doesn't mean passive aggressiveness or retaliation. To clarify: I don't mean that if he does anything rude or disrespectful to you, you can't get angry with him. If he's hurting your feelings or doing something that upsets, you're asking him!

But tell him the keyword in that expression. Don't get mad about him and try to hurt him because he's bothering you, and don't say to him that when you're seething inside, everything's' right.' Give him the room, to be honest with you, be honest with him.

People are only dishonest when telling someone the truth is not comfortable. When you teach him that he can be confident telling you the truth, even if you don't want to hear it, he will always be honest with you.

If he feels safe to tell you whatever he wants, it establishes a deep bond between you that is very hard to break. It is one of the most significant strong, lasting love building blocks.

3. Make sure You're Speaking the Same ' Love Language':

People differently show love and receive love. If he wants love to be received in a different way than you want to show it, then he might feel like he receives no love from you.

This is a basic understanding because when you realize that people like to accept and receiving love in various ways can reveal to you the source of the problems you might have had in your relationships.

The other main idea is that people like getting love just as they want to show respect.

Which means if he likes to show you love by sending you thoughtful gifts, by accepting thoughtful gifts, he also wants to receive love.

If you're trying to show him love with kind words, it's not going to be as meaningful to him as if you were giving him a thoughtful gift because you wouldn't speak his language of love.

Just try to show him love the way he wants to show you love, and you will feel much more loved and appreciated. That, in effect, would kindle and deepen his love for you.

4. Match His Commitment Degree to You Don't Chase After His Love:

Some people usually commit the mistake of assuming that if they act like they are in a serious, committed relationship, they're going to wake up and want to be in a serious, committed relationship. The fact is, this is the exact opposite of how it works, and almost every time, it ends in heartbreak. Here's how guys work: when you encourage him, he won't feel compelled to' lock you down' and fall deeply in love with you.

A way he can be inspired is not to commit himself and act as if you're already in a committed relationship; it's to show him that you are worth it. That you're a catch that anybody would be lucky to have and that if he wants you, he has to' win' you. And how are you doing this? Simple: you suit your relationship level of commitment.

If he doesn't commit to you, you shouldn't commit to him. When you commit to him without any effort from him, it shows him that to have your love; he doesn't have to try hard.

He doesn't have to give you affection; he doesn't have to pledge to you; he doesn't have to put in the effort that you already devote and contribute to him. You're showing him that no matter what effort he puts in; you're going to be there for him.

So you can save your ego-esteem and start forcing him to step up if he wants you by matching his commitment level and trying to commit to this only if he did commit to you.

And you want him to love you; the safest way is to give him a natural urge to step up and win you.'

To inspire him by not devoting yourself to him unless he's "locked you down" explicitly and devoted himself to you. They make him work harder to keep them and fall in love with you quicker by maintaining your self-respect and freedom until he says that he wants a serious, committed relationship.

5. Have Your Own Fulfilling Life Outside Relationship:

One enormous reality regarding useful links is they can't be all. We must be part of a happy life, not the whole thing.

You both need to enjoy your own lives even if you're not together. Being so wrapped in one another that you are the only source of happiness for each other is a formula for co-dependency, tension, and a toxic relationship.

Make sure you let him have his own life just as outside the relationship you have your personal experience. I like to say that the cake is not a great relationship-it's the icing on top of the cake. The cake should be your outdoor life, and friendship is what puts the icing on top of it and makes it all even better. Once they enter into a relationship, two people should be happy and content with their lives, so they can put their happiness together and share it. The connection is not supposed to be your only source of joy if that is a disaster recipe.

8 Ways to Make Your Man Realize Your Importance

Ladies, you deserve respect for your treatment. You deserve the attention that you need. You need to do something about it if your man begins to ignore you. The last thing you're going to do is breaking up with him. You may want to try to make your boyfriend realize your significance as a partner and as a woman first.

You can do this by:

1. Know your value:

The first thing is, you should know what you deserve to be loved, cared for, and appreciated by your partner. You're unique, don't forget. You're incredible. Rate yourself, therefore. Don't let your boyfriend continue to make you feel you're not an extraordinary person. He's lucky to have you, so he's supposed to treasure you as you cherish him.

2. Tell him what you feel:

Freely talk is the main thing to a healthy and functional relationship. If you begin to feel like he no longer appreciates you as his partner, you need to speak up. Be frank about your feelings. Share your grievances. Be clear about it.

You might not always focus on the negative, however. Emphasize that you tell him all this stuff because you want to continue with your relationship. You want to keep him honest. You're helping your boyfriend understand his faults by expressing your feelings and giving him a chance to make it up to you.

3. Act what you feel:

Sometimes, it's not enough to tell your boyfriend what you think. After your long conversation with him, you may not see any changes, weeks, or even months. He may think he's nothing different about the scenario. Now, let your actions speak to him to make him feel the weight of the matter. Create a small gap. Don't call or text at all times. Don't see him all the time. Do not follow what he says at all times. It will help him realize how serious you are about the problem by giving him the cold shoulder. Not seeing him, too, which will often make him long for you.

Remember, if he loves you, he won't let you continue to feel unloved, unimportant, and unloved. He's going to do it for you. He's going to make you feel relevant again.

4. Go out with your other friends:

Spending time with your friends even when you're in a relationship is always a good thing. You'll feel refreshed when you go out with them. You're going to feel like you're not in a bag.

Now, when your man begins to make you feel less urgent, going out with your friends is even more helpful. Let him see that with your mates, you're having fun. Show him that he doesn't just depend on your happiness. He may only realize that without him, he cannot afford to see you become accustomed to living.

5. Limit the stuff you're doing for him at all times:

Always cook for him? Give him a massage at all times? Every time you fight, are you still the one who makes peace with him? Are you always the one who says that you're sorry, even if he's the one to blame? He may be too accustomed to seeing you still be there for him and being in love with him head over heels that he no longer understands how vital your role is in his life.

To stop this, make sure you restrict the things you're doing for him at all times. Yeah, do not hesitate, do not stop. When you stop doing the things you used to do for him, it may make him feel you don't care for him anymore, so let him know your value just enough.

6. Show how independent you are:

One of the best ways to make your boyfriend understand that it is essential to show him how strong and independent you are. To love him is not to make him your world. Show him that the things you like to do can still be done without him. Travel by yourself. Go to work on your own. Eat by yourself. Watch a movie on its own. Do all things related to you on your own will make him realize he's not the only source of energy that will power your life.

7. Moderate your tolerance:

If you're too tolerant of what he's doing, even if you don't like it, then he'll think he's doing nothing wrong. He's going to continue doing this his way. Also, it will be too easy for him to stop seeing your importance if he thinks he has full control over things and you.

Moderate the sensitivity, therefore. Stand up on your ground. Know when to let him do some things and know when not to let him do any things.

8. Check your yeses:

In connection with the previous tip, your boyfriend might be too complacent if you give in to whatever he wants. He's not going to take you seriously. So, never be that kind of girlfriend of yes. Instead, watch your yeses and learn to say no if necessary. Not to offer him to treat you less.

You could say you don't have to make an effort to make people see your importance. However, you don't just get out without trying to fix it when you're in an unhealthy relationship. If he doesn't know the value, you may want to make him realize how lucky he's got you. So, if he keeps ignoring you and doesn't consider you as his girl, you know what to do.

10 Tips to keep Him, completely in Love with You Just He wishes to be your superhero— so let him do it.

1.Infidelity in relationships is a major concern.

It's important to figure out why men cheat (as well as how to keep your man from doing it to you), whether you've been cheated on before or trying to avoid it from ever happening.

Many people are not lying because they no longer love you. Men cheat in their sex lives because they want more variety.

Many men complain that they're bored. We want their friends to feel adored. We want their rights to be recognized. They're sick of deceiving you.

They want a partner that puts them at the center of their lives, and they no longer feel yours as a priority.

Sometimes it's because you speak different languages of love, and some men say that procreating with as many women as possible for the species ' survival is a biological order.

Whatever the cause, people have an inherent need for their partners to feel respected and appreciated. It is most disconcerting for a man to know that in some way he has misled his partner. He would like to be her protector.

So, here's the way to keep your guy (and you alone) in love with you and keep him from cheating: 1. Be prepared to initiate sex.

Men are contrasting gender with desirability. Help your man feel desired by physically expressing your love.

2. Be open to experimenting.

Getting comfortable can be simple, and fear of the unknown will stop you from being open to various sexual experiences.

Let your man try with you new things. If you don't, someone else's going to be there.

I'm not saying you're repulsive to engage in sexual activity, but let the man you love to experience new things.

3. Don't be too welcoming.

Sometimes a woman may become too accommodating in a relationship.

Men have a very clear picture of what a lifetime partner looks like, and this is often in sharp contrast to whom he may have briefly met. Women work to become the person they want to be their friend, and they lose themselves in doing so. One day, their guy knows he's asking for this, but he's not sure it's what he wants.

Continue your friendship with a good sense of self.

4. Don't get too much control.

Often without knowing it, we try to control the other person to do what works best for us when we get into relationships.

They indulge in destructive habits in relationships such as moaning, accusing, questioning, nagging, intimidating, punishing, bribing, or manipulating.

5. Make sure he knows how much he loves you.

Often they start to get a false sense of security when women get the guy and get engaged. Note, it is voluntary for all partnerships.

At any moment, a person can leave. With this country's divorce rate, we need to note how important it is to have a positive relationship, not just to get one.

6. Let him have his own time.

Many men cheat because the relationship is starting to hemmed-in. Engaging in an affair will give them a sense of independence in a marriage that they lose.

Without you, let your man have time for himself. Don't want to monopolize the entire time of your man. To spend with family, pursue hobbies, etc., be open to time apart, so he doesn't feel free.

7. Be mindful of your feelings.

If we know it or not, women are experts in using their feelings to express volumes without any words. We express our partners ' frustration, rage, sorrow, and disappointment.

Some men start looking for another companion to idolatry them the way you used to. Do not forget, your man wants to know that he is dazzling you, not that he is continually failing you.

8. Consider your partnership a priority.

Sometimes, when a man cheats, you can find that the woman also has a non-sexual affair. It's more appropriate socially.

This adultery takes the form of giving priority over the relationship to something— something. This could be a job, kids, a sick relative, a charity, or anything that puts her man lower than the first position on her totem pole.

Prioritize your friendship above all else. This is the relationship that you want to last for your entire life. Some aspects will fade away, and if you consciously continue to do so, the connection will still be there.

9. Learn the language of passion.

Learn the language of love for your man and speak it daily to him. He's going to know that he's loved and stay true to you.

10. That's right. Find the pattern of his partnership.

I don't know how to fight the debate about biology. Some men just believe that having sex with as many women as they can be hard-wired into their genes.

If this is your guy, what you do probably doesn't matter. Try to recognize these people by talking about their experience of dating early on.

If this is your man's pattern, he probably won't change because you love him best. Discrimination at the start is your best defense against this issue.

Don't point your finger at your friend if you're upset with your marriage. Look into the mirror and assess what the unhappiness triggers.

If you want your guy to have something special, ask for it. If he gives you everything you want, then it's great! If he doesn't, then look for the solution inside of you.

Consider your man as he is and learn to handle your relationship better. And if he violates one of your non-negotiables, your best option might be to quit.

7 Sweet & Easy Secrets to Love Your Man

1. Compliment him.

Where did we get the impression that only women like to be told that they look good, that they smell good, that they are hot, smart, or sexy?

In my childhood, I had the impression that guys are smarter than women for their looks and sex appeal. Guys shouldn't worry about things like what clothes they're wearing or if their new haircut looks good, right?

2. Tell him that you appreciate what he and your parents are doing for you.

If your partner is working outside the home, let him know you support what he is doing. Even if he loves his job, I promise that when he thinks of throwing in the towel or shouting at his manager or just sitting in his office all day, there are days. But he's not doing that. You and your family may be part of the reason.

Breadwinning is an incredible responsibility for any human, and for men, it is even more emphasized by society. Sadly, their earning potential in our culture is often linked to their quality. As bad as that may be, it only gets worse if we don't understand that people are under stress and their commitment.

If your partner works with the children at home, he sacrifices for your family as well. Just as he undoubtedly enjoys being the parent at home and takes immense joy in it, all parents have moments when they too want to throw in the towel (or diaper), yell at the boss (the baby?), or hide in a corner. But they're not! They're in there, elbow-deep in something yucky, and taking care of the kids throughout the day.

It's easy: tell him you know how difficult it can be to do what he's doing. Tell him that you appreciate it and see his dedication. It's not about the money — your or his — it's about understanding something that is typically taken for granted by society.

3. Make time to get warm in the bedroom for stuff.

No, he's certainly not a sex god, but for both of you, the best sex feels transcendent, reciprocal, connected, steamy, and dreamy. Making him feel like the diet of your own private species, and reciprocating him, is likely to make your two lives happier.

No one ever owes their partner sex, but in a healthy relationship, fostering attraction is a good thing. If slipping into the role of sex-god or goddess when you're at home is hard, try in a hotel room for a night. If that's out of your range, you can also have fun in a tent in the woods. You can even chat about fantasies at home or watch sexy pictures together or take some of your own boudoir photos. Don't feel like revealing your entire body or becoming too racious? Try to take close-ups of a sexy part of the body, but not so clear. Your bra belt on your back, your undies at the tip of the thigh, peeking out of your jeans. There are plenty of design suggestions out there.

It's easy: feed your desire for him. Choose to fantasize about him, about a time you've been together, about that body's favorite part you love so much. So pile up on him all that you want when you have the next chance to be alone together.

4. Be in support of his time alone.

I'm going to be honest, for me, this one was the toughest. I don't know why, but when Ivan and I first came together, I was concerned about how much time he spent surfing or riding his mountain bike. We both played, we didn't see each other a lot, and I felt as though I had been thrown away.

That was a lot of pressure and not very fair to place on my father. We finally learned how to plan our time alone— and I took advantage of being so tolerant of my need to work out, write, or just read a book in bed.

Unless he's so lost in his time alone that you're absent from his thoughts, it's a good thing to be separated! If you're concerned about the length of time he's going to be home, just set a time when he's going to be back and prepare later together. Being apart will give you more to think about, and if he uses his time alone for exercise or relaxation, he is likely to be happier and healthier for doing it.

It's easy: Smile when he says he's going to do things on his own that makes him happy. Give a kiss to him. He should know that he has been noticed, understood, and helped.

5. Put your phone down.

I'm just as guilty as anybody else. There's always one more message, one more friend's text, another emergency work emergency arising. But you have to put down the phone and see the guy in front of you.

I try to take a deep breath when I get caught in this loop and remember the worst thing that could happen if I miss anything that buzzes at me. He knows, of course, if it's a real emergency, but most things can wait.

I still see him there when I put down my phone and look at his face. I see the man I love, the man I met so many years ago, and I think how ridiculous it is that I don't get involved with him.

Make a deal with your partner: in just a few terms, if you need to pick up your phone for something urgent, let the other one know what it is. "The server is down," or "the sitter is calling," is a justifiable reason to step away for a moment, but let him know why you're doing it, and you're going to be back.

It's easy: be with the person you love at the moment you're with. Try not to let it slip away while you're looking at a screen.

6. Look in the eyes of him.

You don't have to gaze at each other longingly as you used to at the roller rink with your boyfriend of 9th grade. Only take a moment to interact with each other, eye-to-eye, and share the looks.

Unless you listened to assumptions about what guys want, you wouldn't think it would be on his list of good things to have a soul-looking link, but I suggest you try it. With a smile or a friendly gesture, look at him in the eye and hold his gaze for three seconds. It's a flirting tactic that works with individuals as it makes the other person feel like the only one in the house. He may now be your boyfriend or husband, but he still deserves a special feeling.

Conclusion:

People relate to an attitude shaped by previous experiences. One learns from the experience, and earlier partners ' negative actions affect their conduct with a new partner. Every woman wants an ideal man for the commitment that is in line with her desires, and when she meets him, she wants to continue to have a relationship with him. Once a relationship becomes a commitment, the unwillingness to face emotional pain must be put aside. It is necessary to consider a severe bond as a fresh start.

Commitment is the most important thing in a relationship. After reading this guide, you are able to understand the real meaning of lifetime commitment. It may help you to find out the ideal man as your partner for a lifetime commitment. You can learn how to keep your man in love with you. And the most important thing is that the person you are in love with or in a relationship, also feeling the same for you, is he is really committed to you or not? After reading this guide, you are able to find out the right person you want in your life with whom you spend your life happily.

However, you know your perspectives, and whatever words you choose to use, we hope you will find the information helpful in this book when considering different care and support choices.

References:

In love with someone derived from:

https://www.bolde.com/8-differences-loving-someone-being-in-love/

Ideal Man for life time derived from:

https://omoleye90.wordpress.com/2013/02/18/an-ideal-man/

Qualities and characteristics of ideal man derived from:

https://www.psychalive.org/seven-qualities-of-an-ideal-partner/

https://www.uckg.org/the-5-qualities-of-an-ideal-man/

How love changes a person life is derived from:

https://www.canopyhealth.com/en/members/articles/how-does-love-affect-our-physical-health.html

https://www.theodysseyonline.com/life-changes-love-someone

Life time Commitment is derived from:

https://www.123helpme.com/commitment-to-a-partner-preview.asp?id=198164

https://freespiritcentre.ca/what-does-commitment-really-mean/

https://www.accountabilitycoach.com/what-does-commitment-mean-to-you/

Ideal Partner is derived from:

https://www.psychalive.org/dating-resolutions-7-characteristics-of-an-ideal-partner/

How to find he is committed to you or not? Is derived from:

https://www.elitedaily.com/dating/signs-he-is-committed-to-you/2021907

https://www.thetalko.com/hell-only-do-these-15-things-if-hes-committed-to-only-you/

https://www.psychologytoday.com/us/blog/sliding-vs-deciding/201707/3-true-signs-relationship-commitment

http://www.lovedatingdoc.com/10-signs-he-loves-you/

Best Words About Love, Commitment and Relationship is derived from:

https://lifehacks.io/inspirational-love-quotes-sayings/

https://www.goodreads.com/quotes/tag/perfect-man

https://www.brainyquote.com/topics/ideal-man-quotes

How to keep your man is derived from?

https://inspiringtips.com/how-to-keep-a-man/